Ob/Gyn Sonog

A REVIEW FOR THE REGISTRY EXAM

Ob/Gyn Sonography Review

A REVIEW FOR THE ARDMS OBSTETRICS & GYNECOLOGY EXAM

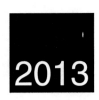

2013

Kathryn A. Gill, MS, RT, RDMS
Institute of Ultrasound Diagnostics
Daphne, Alabama

Misty H. Sliman, RT, RDMS
Institute of Ultrasound Diagnostics
Daphne, Alabama

Peter W. Callen, MD
UCSF School of Medicine
San Francisco, California

Editor in Chief

Davies Publishing, Inc.
32 South Raymond Avenue
Pasadena, California 91105-1935
Phone 626-792-3046
Facsimile 626-792-5308
e-mail info@daviespublishing.com
www.daviespublishing.com

Printed and bound in the United States of America

Library of Congress Cataloging-in-Publication Data

Gill, Kathryn A.
OB/GYN sonography review : a review for the ARDMS obstetrics & gynecology exam, 2002-2003 / Kathryn A. Gill, Misty H. Sliman, Peter W. Callen.
p. ; cm.
Includes bibliographical references.
ISBN 0-941022-53-6
Ultrasonics in obstetrics—Examinations, questions, etc. I. Sliman, Misty H. II. Callen, Peter W. III. Title.
[DNLM: 1. obstetrics—Examination Questions. 2. Genital Diseases, Female—ultrasonography—Examination questions. 3. Pregnancy Complications—ultrasonography—Examination Questions. WQ 18.2 G475o 2003]
RG527.5.U48G55 2003
618.2'07543'076—dc21

2002041681

Preface

THIS MOCK EXAM is a question/answer/reference review of ob/gyn sonography for those RDMS candidates who plan to take the ARDMS Obstetrics and Gynecology specialty examination. It is designed as an adjunct to your regular study and as a method to help you determine your strengths and weaknesses so that you can study more effectively. *Ob/Gyn Sonography Review* covers everything on the current ARDMS exam content outline and in fact follows that outline, which you will find in Part VI of this book.

Facts about *Ob/Gyn Sonography Review*:

- It precisely covers and follows the current ARDMS exam outline.

- It focuses exclusively on the Obstetrics and Gynecology specialty exam to ensure thorough coverage of even the smallest subtopic on the exam. (For the Ultrasound Physics and Instrumentation exam, see *Ultrasound Physics Review*.)

- Topics are covered to the same extent as on the exam itself. Subject headings include the approximate percentage of the exam that a particular topic represents so you know the relative importance of each topic and can study more effectively.

- *Ob/Gyn Sonography Review* contains more than 515 questions, many of which are image-based or otherwise illustrated.

- Explanations are clear and conveniently referenced for fact-checking or further study.

- Each section is keyed to the ARDMS exam outline so that you always know where you are, what you are studying, and how it applies to your preparation.

- A bibliography appears at the end of the book, as does the exam outline and contact information for the ARDMS.

Ob/Gyn Sonography Review effectively simulates content and experience of the exam. Current ARDMS standards call for approximately 170 multiple-choice questions to be answered during a three-hour period. That is, you will have an average time of 1 minute to answer each question. A passing score is between 65% and 75%, depending on the difficulty of the particular exam. Timing your practice sessions according to the number of questions you need to finish will help you prepare for the pressure experienced by RDMS candidates taking this exam. It also helps to ensure that your score accurately reflects your strengths and weaknesses so that you study more efficiently and with greater purpose in the limited time you can devote to preparation. Because the content of this

Q&A review is formatted and weighted according to the registry's outline of topics and subtopics, you can readily identify those areas on which you should concentrate.

We include below and strongly recommend that you read *Taking and Passing Your Exam*, by Don Ridgway, RVT, who offers useful tips and practical strategies for taking and passing the ARDMS examinations.

Finally, you have not only our best wishes for success, but also our admiration for taking this big and important step in your career.

Kathy Gill

Kathryn A. Gill, MS, RT, RDMS
Daphne, Alabama

Taking and Passing Your Exam

by Don Ridgway, RVT[*]

Preparing for your exam . . .

Study. And then study some more. Knowing your stuff is the most important factor in your success. Start early, set a regular study schedule, and stick to it. Make your schedule specific so you know exactly what to study on a particular day. Write it down. Establish realistic goals so that you don't build a mountain you can't climb.

As to *what* you study, don't just read aimlessly. Focus your efforts on what you need to know. Rely on a core group of dependable references, referring to others as necessary to firm up your understanding of specific topics. Let the ARDMS exam outlines guide you. And use different but complementary study methods—texts, flashcards, and mock exams—to exercise those neural pathways.

Ease down on studying the week before. Wind down, reduce stress, build confidence, and rest up. Don't cram! And no studying the night before. You had your chance. Watch a movie, relax, go to bed early, and sleep well.

Organize your things the night before. Lay out comfortable clothes (including a sweater or sweatshirt in case the testing center is cold), pencils, your ARDMS test-admission papers, car and house keys, glasses, prescriptions, directions to the test center, and any other personal items you might need. Be prepared!

The day of your exam . . .

Eat lightly. You do not want to fall asleep during the exam. Go easy on the coffee or tea so your bladder doesn't distract you halfway through the exam.

Arrive early. Plan to arrive at the test center early, especially if you haven't been there before. Take directions, including the telephone number of the testing center in case you have to make contact en route. You don't need a wrong-offramp adventure.

Be confident. As you wait for the exam to begin, smile, lift both hands, wave them toward yourself, and say, "Bring it on."

---

[*] Don Ridgway is the author of *Introduction to Vascular Scanning: A Guide for the Complete Beginner* and editor of *Vascular Technology Review 2003.* Don teaches and practices at Grossmont College and Hospital in El Cajon, California.

During the exam . . .

Read each question twice before answering. Guess how easy it is to get one word wrong and misunderstand the whole question.

Try to answer the question before looking at the choices. Formulating an answer before peeking at the possibilities minimizes the distractibility of the incorrect answer choices, which in the test-making business are called—guess what!—*distractors.*

Knock off the easy ones first. First answer the questions you feel good about. Then go back for the more difficult items. Next, attack the really tough ones. Taking notes on long or tricky questions often can jog your memory or put the question in new light. For questions you just cannot answer with certainty, eliminate the obviously wrong answer choices and then guess.

Guessing. Passing the exam depends on the number of correct answers you make. Because unanswered questions are counted as *in*correct, it makes sense to guess when all else fails. The ARDMS itself advises that "it is to the candidate's advantage to answer all possible questions." Guessing alone improves your chances of scoring a point from 0 (for an unanswered question) to 20% (for randomly picking one of five possible answers). Eliminating answer choices you know or suspect are wrong further improves your odds of success. By using your knowledge and skill to eliminate three of the five answer choices before guessing, for example, you increase your odds of scoring a point to 50%.

Don't second-guess. The common wisdom is that your first answer is more likely than revised answers to be correct. Actual studies indicate that when you return to a question and change the answer, you'll probably be wrong. Change an answer only if you're quite sure you should.

Pace yourself; watch the time. Work methodically and quickly to answer those you know, and make your best guesses at the gnarly ones. Leave no question unanswered.

Don't despair 50 minutes into the exam. At some point you may feel that things just aren't going well. Take 10 seconds to breathe deeply—in for a count of five, out for a count of five. Relax. Recall that you need only about three out of four correct answers to pass. If you've prepared reasonably well, a passing score is attainable even if you feel sweat running down your back.

Taking the exam on computer . . .

Some candidates express concern about taking the registry exam on computer. Most folks find this to be pretty easy; some find it off-putting, at least in prospect. But the computerized exams are quite convenient: You can take the exam at your convenience (a far cry from the days of one exam per year), you know whether or not you passed before you leave the testing center (compare that to waiting weeks and even months, as used to be the case), and you can reschedule the exam after 90 days if you happen not to pass the first time (rather than waiting another six months to a year). Another good point: The illustrations are said to be clearer on computer than in the booklets at a Scantron-type exam.

Taking the test by computer is not complicated. The center even gives you a tutorial to be sure you know what you need to do. You sit in a carrel with a computer and answer the multiple-choice questions by pointing and clicking with a mouse. There is a clock on the display letting you know how much time is left. Use it to pace yourself. Scratch paper is available; make liberal use of it.

You can mark questions to return for answering later. A display shows which questions have not been answered so you can return to them. When you have finished, you click on "DONE," and you find out immediately whether you passed.

It's nothing to be afraid of. The principles are the same as those for any exam. Be methodical and keep breathing.

Summary . . .

Preparing for the exam:
- Study
- Use flashcards
- Join a study group
- Wind down a week before
- Don't cram
- Relax!

The day of your exam:
- Eat lightly, arrive early, avoid coffee
- Arrive early
- Take a sweater
- Be confident!

During the exam:

- Read each question twice
- Answer the question before looking at the answer choices
- Answer the easy ones first
- Guess when necessary
- Don't second-guess your first answers
- Pace yourself
- Don't despair

Taking the exam on computer:

- Just point and click
- Take notes
- Mark and return to the hard questions
- Use the on-screen clock to pace yourself
- Be methodical
- Breathe!

Contents

Other

PART I

Obstetrics

First Trimester
Second/Third Trimester (Normal Anatomy)
Placenta
Assessment of Gestational Age
Complications
Amniotic Fluid
Genetic Studies
Fetal Demise
Fetal Abnormalities
Coexisting Disorders

FIRST TRIMESTER [6–8%]

Gestational sac

Yolk sac

Embryo (normal physiologic development/sonographic appearance)

Ovaries (corpus luteum)

Cul-de-sac

Pregnancy failure

Ectopic pregnancy

1. The pelvic mass most commonly seen during a normal first trimester pregnancy is:

    A. Leiomyoma
    B. Cystic teratoma
    C. Corpus luteal cyst
    D. Theca lutein cysts
    E. Cystadenoma

2. The primitive hindbrain can be seen as a cystic structure within the embryonic head. It is called the:

    A. Diencephalons
    B. Rhombencephalon
    C. Prosencephalon

D. Mesencephalon

E. Encephalocele

3. The maternal side of the developing placenta is referred to as the:

 A. Decidua basalis

 B. Decidua capsularis

 C. Decidua vera

 D. Decidua parietalis

 E. Decidua chorion

4. Up to 10 weeks gestational age, the mean diameter of the normal gestational sac should grow:

 A. 0.5 mm/day

 B. 1 mm/day

 C. 2 mm/day

 D. 3 mm/day

 E. 4 mm/day

5. Physiologic herniation of fetal intestine outside the fetal abdomen should not be seen after gestational age:

 A. 6 weeks

 B. 8 weeks

 C. 10 weeks

 D. 12 weeks

 E. 14 weeks

6. One should be able to image a normal intrauterine gestational sac transabdominally when the International Reference Preparation (IRP) level for hCG is equal to or greater than:

 A. 1000 units/liter

 B. 1200 units/liter

 C. 1800 units/liter

 D. 2400 units/liter

 E. 3600 units/liter

7. Which of the following is NOT an indication of ectopic pregnancy?

 A. Fluid in the cul-de-sac

 B. Fluid within the endometrial cavity

 C. Double decidual ring

 D. Adnexal mass

 E. Fluid in the right upper quadrant

8. A missed abortion is defined as:

 A. Retention of a dead conceptus for a prolonged period (e.g., 2 months)

 B. Retention of products of conception with bleeding

    C. Blighted ovum without bleeding
    D. Blighted ovum with bleeding
    E. Ectopic pregnancy without bleeding

9.   All of the following characteristics suggest an <u>abnormal</u> early pregnancy EXCEPT:

    A. Irregular sac shape
    B. Poor decidual ring
    C. Dilated cervix
    D. Fundal implantation
    E. Fluid around the sac

10.   Your patient is 10 weeks by good menstrual dates but presents with pregnancy-induced hypertension. You suspect:

    A. Threatened abortion
    B. Hydatidiform mole
    C. Normal pregnancy
    D. Ectopic pregnancy
    E. Blighted ovum

11.   Your patient has a positive pregnancy test and presents with bleeding and cramping. Of the following sonographic findings, which one would make you suspect an inevitable abortion?

    A. Low implantation
    B. Irregular sac shape
    C. Poor decidual reaction
    D. Double yolk sac
    E. Dilated cervix

12.   A *heterotopic* pregnancy is:

    A. An abdominal ectopic pregnancy
    B. An ectopic pregnancy with a normal intrauterine pregnancy
    C. A twin ectopic pregnancy
    D. A cervical ectopic pregnancy
    E. A fertility-assisted pregnancy

13.   To differentiate an early intrauterine pregnancy from a pseudogestational sac, it helps to visualize the:

    A. Decidualized endometrium
    B. Chorionic villi
    C. Yolk sac
    D. Vitelline duct
    E. Corpus luteal cyst

14.   A yolk sac is considered abnormal when its diameter exceeds:

    A. 2 mm

B. 3 mm

C. 4 mm

D. 5 mm

E. 6 mm

15. Which of these drugs may be used to treat an early unruptured ectopic pregnancy in order to preserve fertility?

A. Thalidomide

B. Methotrexate

C. Diethylstilbestrol (DES)

D. Pergonal

E. Danazol

This transvaginal image applies to questions 16 and 17.

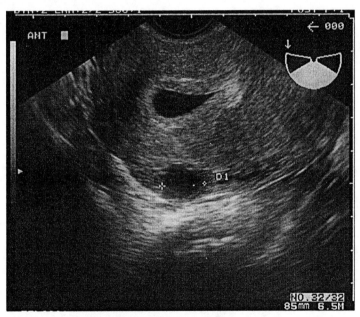

16. This sagittal transvaginal image demonstrates a normal appearing intrauterine gestational sac. The hypoechoic structure indicated by the calipers most likely represents a(n):

A. Leiomyoma

B. Engorged vessel

C. Cyst

D. Artifact

E. Ovary

17. The previous image shows the uterine position to be:

A. Levoposed

B. Dextroposed
C. Anteflexed
D. Retroflexed
E. Unidentifiable

> This transverse image applies to
> questions 18–21.

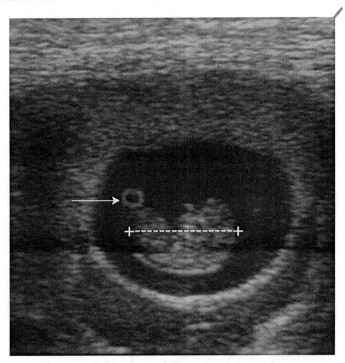

18. A patient presents with a positive pregnancy test and bright red spotting. By dates she is 8–9 weeks. What does this transverse image demonstrate?

    A. An anembryonic pregnancy
    B. Subchorionic hemorrhage
    C. Placental abruption
    D. Normal amnion
    E. Second gestational sac

19. What is being measured in this image?

    A. Gestational sac
    B. Embryonic disc
    C. Crown-rump length
    D. Biparietal diameter
    E. Abdominal circumference

20. To what is the arrow pointing?

    A. Gestational sac
    B. Fetal head

C. Amniotic cyst

D. Yolk sac

E. Umbilical cord

21. Your patient relates a history of amenorrhea for 7 weeks. Her home pregnancy test was negative, but her serum beta-hCG exceeds 4000. What does this image demonstrate?

A. Normal empty uterus with periovulatory endometrium

B. Normal early intrauterine pregnancy

C. Fluid contained within the endometrial cavity

D. Pseudocyesis with an endometrial cyst

E. Degenerating submucosal fibroid

22. In a ruptured ectopic pregnancy, which section of the fallopian tube is potentially the most life-threatening?

A. Interstitial

B. Ampulla

C. Isthmus

D. Fimbria

E. Ligamentous

23. The *double bleb sign* refers to the sonographic presentation of:

A. The amnion and chorion

B. Two intrauterine gestational sacs

C. The amnion and yolk sac

D. A heterotopic pregnancy

E. A bicornuate uterus

24. This patient is 10 weeks by good menstrual dates, but her doctor feels that she is small for gestational age and he cannot hear any fetal heart tones. He orders a sonogram to confirm viability. An M-mode was not included. Referring to the image on the following page, what do you suspect?

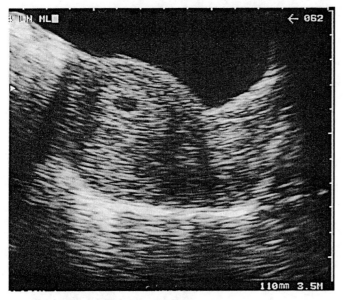

A. She has an ectopic pregnancy.
B. The sac is too large for the embryo/fetus inside, suggesting an abnormal pregnancy.
C. The sac is too small for a 10 week gestation, suggesting incorrect dates.
D. There are two sacs of about 5 weeks size, suggesting twins.
E. She is not really pregnant, suggesting pseudocyesis.

25. To what is the arrow pointing?

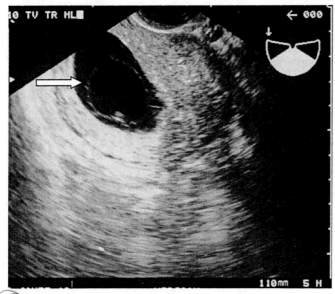

A. Amnion
B. Chorion
C. Yolk sac
D. Septum
E. Synechia

26. All of the following are associated with trophoblastic disease EXCEPT:

    A. Theca lutein cysts
    B. Pregnancy-induced hypertension
    C. Hyperemesis gravidarum
    D. Large for gestational age
    E. Normal fetus

27. Of the following methods of calculating an estimated date of confinement (EDC), which is the most reliable?

    A. Sac measurement
    B. Crown rump length
    C. First sign of quickening
    D. Fundal height of uterus
    E. McDonald's measurement

28. Because of spinal segmentation, crown-rump length measurements begin to lose accuracy after how many gestational weeks?

    A. 3
    B. 5
    C. 7
    D. 9
    E. 11

29. In this image of a first trimester pregnancy the arrow is pointing to:

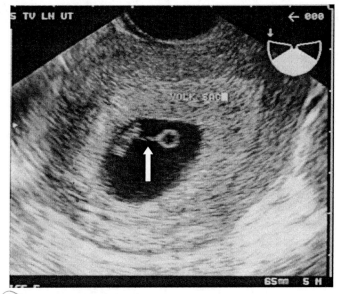

    A. Vitelline duct
    B. Umbilical cord
    C. Ductus venosus
    D. Amniotic band
    E. Synechia

30. What is being measured in this 11-week fetus?

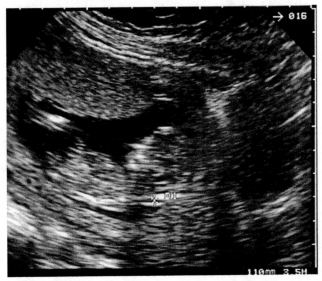

A. Nuchal fold
B. Nuchal translucency
C. Cervical cord
D. Cervical spine
E. Amniochorio separation

31. What is the significance of the above measurement?

A. It is a good indicator of gestational age.
B. It is a good indicator of possible placenta abruption.
C. It is a good indicator of possible chromosomal abnormalities.
D. It is an indicator of possible neural tube defects.
E. It is of no practical significance.

32. A longitudinal image shows an intrauterine gestational sac that occupies 1/2 of the uterine cavity. The sac size indicates that the gestational age of the pregnancy should be:

A. 4 weeks
B. 6 weeks
C. 8 weeks
D. 10 weeks
E. 12 weeks

33. A patient presents with a positive pregnancy test, bleeding, and cramping. The sonogram reveals an intrauterine gestational sac containing an echogenic structure but no heartbeat. Measurement of the structure shows it to be 11 mm in length. The most likely diagnosis is:

A. Partial mole
B. Missed abortion

C. Blighted ovum
D. Early pregnancy failure
E. Placenta previa

34. Which of the following procedures would be performed to treat the incompetent cervix?

A. Shirodkar
B. McDonald's procedure
C. Cone procedure
D. A and B
E. A and C

35. Which statement about ectopic pregnancies is NOT true?

A. The most common clinical symptom is pain.
B. If a patient has had a previous ectopic pregnancy, she is at increased risk for a recurrent ectopic pregnancy.
C. Interstitial ectopics are more serious than those located in the ampulla.
D. The increased incidence of ectopic pregnancies is mostly attributable to sexually transmitted diseases.
E. The ovary is the second most common site for ectopic pregnancy

36. Normally, nuchal translucency does not exceed:

A. 1 mm
B. 2 mm
C. 3 mm
D. 4 mm
E. 6 mm

SECOND / THIRD TRIMESTER (NORMAL ANATOMY) [8–12%]

Cranial

Spine

Heart

Thorax

Abdomen (gastrointestinal, genitourinary, general)

Extremities

Fetal position

Other

37. Which best describes the location of the choroid plexus?

A. Within the posterior portion of the fetal brain just inferior to the cerebellum

     B. Within the atria of the lateral ventricles bilaterally

     C. Between the thalami bilaterally

     D. In the most inferior portion of the fetal brain adjacent to the lateral ventricles

     E. At the level of the falx and periventricular vasculature

38. In ruling out hydrocephalus, where would one first begin to see enlargement?

     A. Cisterna magna

     B. Third ventricle

     C. Anterior horns of the lateral ventricles

     D. Lateral ventricular atria

     E. Posterior fossa

> **The following image applies to questions 39 and 40.**

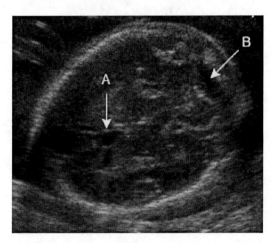

39. What is being documented at label *A* in this image?

     A. Cavum septum pellucidum

     B. Corpus callosum

     C. Cisterna magna

     D. Peduncles

     E. Cerebellum

40. In the same image, what does *B* represent?

     A. 4th ventricle

     B. Thalami

     C. Cisterna magna

     D. Peduncles

     E. Lateral ventricles

41. Normal measurements for the lateral ventricle of the fetal brain are:

     A. 1 mm in the largest dimension transversely

     B. 10 mm in the largest dimension longitudinally

C. 1 cm in the largest dimension <u>transversely</u>
D. 1 cm in the largest dimension longitudinally
E. B and D

42. The landmark used to localize the correct level for measuring fetal biparietal diameter (BPD) and head circumference (HC) is the:

A. Cerebellum
B. Thalami
C. Lateral ventricles
D. Peduncles
E. Cisterna magna

43. What is the arrow pointing to in this transverse image of the fetal head?

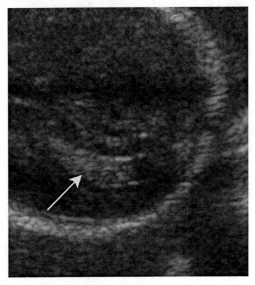

A. Cerebellum
B. Choroid plexus
C. Thalami
D. Cisterna magna
E. Third ventricle

The image on the following page applies to questions 44 and 45.

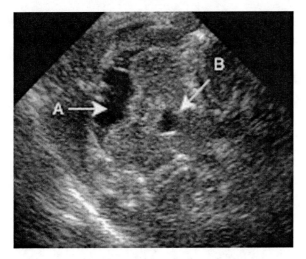

44. The arrow labeled *A* is pointing to:

    A. Vallecula
    B. Tentorium
    C. Posterior fossa
    D. Anterior fossa
    E. Posterior ridge

45. In the same image, *B* represents:

    A. Cisterna magna
    B. Faux
    C. 4th ventricle
    D. Thalami
    E. 3rd ventricle

46. The arrows in this image point to:

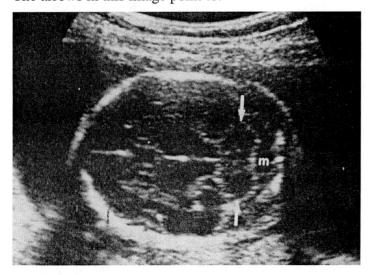

    A. Thalami
    B. Ventricles
    C. Cerebellum
    D. Cavum septum pellucidum

E. Cisterna magna

47. Longitudinal and transverse views of the fetal spine are routine on fetal exam. When the normal fetal spine is imaged transversely, the sonogram demonstrates:

   A. Two ossification centers positioned an equal distance apart and tapering toward the sacrum
   B. Two ossification centers positioned an equal distance apart and splaying outward at the level of the sacrum
   C. Three ossification centers, two posterior and one anterior, with the two posterior centers pointing away from each other
   D. Three ossification centers, two posterior and one anterior, with the two posterior centers pointing toward each other
   E. Three ossification centers, two anterior and one posterior, with the two posterior centers pointing toward each other

48. What best describes the anatomy demonstrated by the arrows in this longitudinal image of the fetal spine?

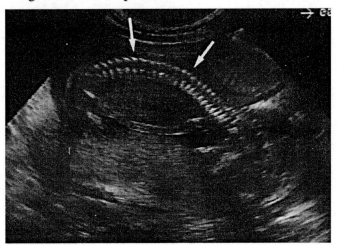

   A. Lamina
   B. Centrum
   C. Transverse process
   D. Pedicles and lamina
   E. Dural sac

The image on the following page applies to questions 49–51.

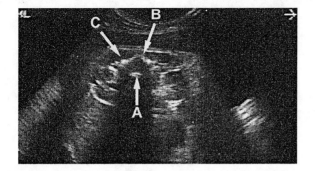

49. In this image, arrow A represents the:

    A. Laminae
    B. Spinal cord
    C. Centrum
    D. Transverse process
    E. Intervertebral disc

50. Arrow B is pointing to the:

    A. Laminae
    B. Spinal cord
    C. Centrum
    D. Spinous process
    E. Intervertebral disc

51. In the same image, to what, specifically, is arrow C pointing?

    A. Laminae
    B. Spinal cord
    C. Centrum
    D. Spinous process
    E. Intervertebral disc

52. What ultrasound modality would you use to prove fetal life on a frozen image?

    A. B-mode
    B. A-mode
    C. M-mode
    D. 3-D
    E. Static scanning

53. Normally, the anatomic structure closest to the spine in a four-chamber view of the fetal heart is the:

    A. Right atrium
    B. Left atrium
    C. Right ventricle
    D. Left ventricle
    E. Apex

54. The fetal heart occupies:

   A. One-fourth of the chest cavity pointing toward the right side of the fetus
   B. One-third of the chest cavity pointing toward the right side of the fetus
   C. One-half of the chest cavity pointing toward the left side of the fetus
   D. One-third of the chest cavity pointing toward the left side of the fetus
   E. One-fourth of the fetal chest cavity medially

55. When examining the fetal heart, the sonographer can rule out 85% of structural heart malformations by imaging the great vessels along with a four-chamber view of the heart. The great vessels consist of the:

   A. RVOT
   B. AVOT
   C. LVOT
   D. A and C
   E. B and C

The following image applies to questions 56–57.

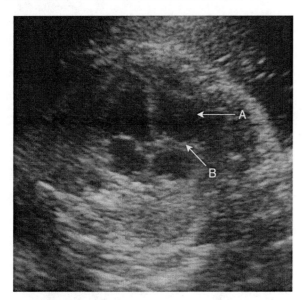

56. In this image the arrow labeled *A* points to the:

   A. Right atrium
   B. Left atrium
   C. Right ventricle
   D. Left ventricle
   E. Ventricular septum

57. In the same image, arrow *B* demonstrates the:

   A. Aortic semilunar valve

B. Pulmonary semilunar valve
C. Tricuspid valve
D. Mitral valve
E. Ventricular septum

58. In a fetal heart, the communication between the right and left atria is termed:

    A. Ventricular septal defect
    B. Atrial septal defect
    C. Atrial orifice
    D. Foramen ovale
    E. Atrial meatus

59. The arrow in this image points to the:

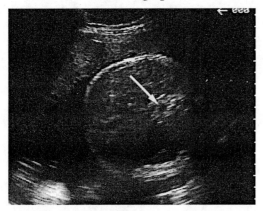

    A. Transverse spine
    B. Transverse diaphragm
    C. Transverse spinal cord
    D. Transverse aorta
    E. Transverse IVC

60. In the body of a normal fetus the heart is positioned at an angle:

    A. 35° to the right of midline
    B. 35° to the left of midline
    C. 45° to the right of midline
    D. 45° to the left of midline
    E. 55° to the left of midline

61. The terms *RVOT* (right ventricular outflow tract) and *LVOT* (left ventricular outflow tract) denote the:

    A. Descending aorta and pulmonary vein
    B. Pulmonary vein and pulmonary artery
    C. Pulmonary artery and ascending aorta
    D. Ascending aorta and inferior vena cava
    E. None of the above

62.   The arrow in this image points to the:

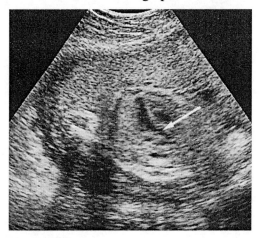

A. RVOT
B. LVOT
C. AORTA
D. IVC
E. AVOT

63.   A small, rounded echogenic structure within the left ventricle of a fetal heart most
likely is:

A. Ventricular septum
B. Aortic semilunar valve
C. Chordae tendineae/papillary muscle
D. Left ventricular embolus
E. CHF

The short-axis view of the fetal heart on the next page applies to questions 64–67.

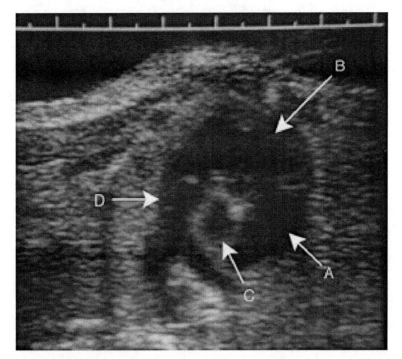

64. What is demonstrated by arrow *A* in this short-axis view of the fetal heart?

    A. Right ventricle
    B. Right atrium
    C. Right ventricular outflow tract
    D. Right pulmonary artery
    E. Aorta

65. Arrow *B* is pointing to:

    A. Right ventricle
    B. Right atrium
    C. Right ventricular outflow tract
    D. Right pulmonary artery
    E. Aorta

66. In the preceding image arrow *C* is pointing to the:

    A. Right ventricle
    B. Right atrium
    C. Right ventricular outflow tract
    D. Right pulmonary artery
    E. Aorta

67. In the same image, the anatomy to which arrow *D* is pointing is best described as the:

    A. Right ventricle
    B. Right atrium
    C. Right ventricular outflow tract

D. Right pulmonary artery

E. Aorta

The following image applies to questions 68–71.

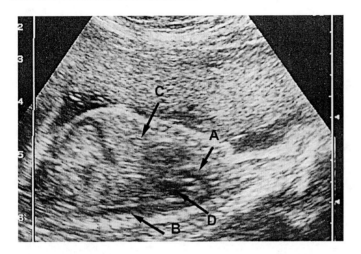

68. Label *A* in this image demonstrates an example of:

A. Left atrium

B. Transverse aorta

C. Ascending aorta

D. Descending aorta

E. Diaphragm

69. In the same image arrow *B* indicates the:

A. Left atrium

B. Transverse aorta

C. Ascending aorta

D. Descending aorta

E. Diaphragm

70. Arrow *C* is pointing to which of the following structures?

A. Left atrium

B. Transverse aorta

C. Ascending aorta

D. Descending aorta

E. Diaphragm

71. Which of the following choices best describes the anatomy represented by *D*?

A. Left atrium

B. Transverse aorta

C. Ascending aorta

    D. Descending aorta
    E. Diaphragm

72. Which of the following views best demonstrates the diaphragm?

    A. Transverse
    B. Oblique to the fetus' left
    C. Four-chamber view of the heart
    D. Oblique to the fetus' right
    E. Coronal

73. Thoracic circumference is measured in the:

    A. True transverse view just below the fetal diaphragm and just above fetal four-chamber heart
    B. True transverse view at the level of fetal four-chamber heart
    C. True longitudinal view at the level of fetal four-chamber heart
    D. Longitudinal view at the level of the diaphragm and just below fetal four-chamber heart
    E. True transverse view just below the fetal diaphragm and at the level of fetal heart motion

74. The candy-cane pulsating vessel imaged somewhat to the left of the spine in a longitudinal scan of the fetus is the:

    A. Descending aorta
    B. Ascending aorta
    C. Ductal arch
    D. Aortic arch
    E. Inferior vena cava

75. This fetal lung (asterisk) is more echogenic than the contralateral lung because of:

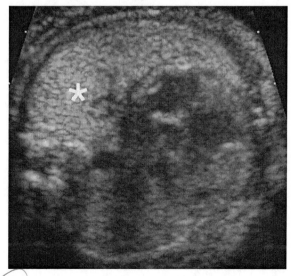

    A. Artifact
    B. Tracheal atresia

C. Fetal lung maturity

D. Congenital diaphragmatic hernia

E. Differential blood flow

76. The fluid-filled stomach should always be visualized in the fetal left upper quadrant. If it is not seen during the course of an exam, one should suspect:

   A. Duodenal atresia

   B. Pyloric stenosis

   C. Esophageal atresia

   D. Jejunoileal obstruction

   E. Ulcerative colitis

77. To what is the arrow pointing in this image?

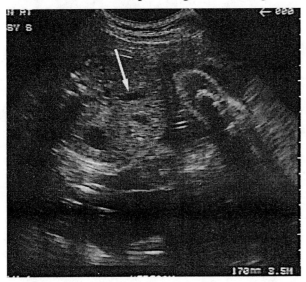

   A. Umbilical vein

   B. Stomach

   C. Hepatic veins

   D. Gallbladder

   E. Portal vein

78. Which of the following provides important prognostic information about fetal renal function?

   A. The presence and evaluation of amniotic fluid by approximately 9 weeks gestation

   B. The presence and evaluation of urine in the fetal bladder and amniotic fluid by approximately 13 weeks gestation

   C. The size of the fetal kidneys

   D. Amniotic fluid volume at term

   E. None of the above

79. The fetal kidneys are most commonly located:

   A. At the level and posterior to the cord insertion

B. Slightly superior and adjacent to the fetal stomach
C. Adjacent to the fetal spine bilaterally
D. Adjacent and inferior to the cord insertion
E. At the level and posterior to the fetal diaphragm

80. The fetal bladder should fill and then empty again approximately every:

    A. 5–10 minutes
    B. 10–15 minutes
    C. 30–45 minutes
    D. 60–75 minutes
    E. 120 minutes

81. What is demonstrated in this image?

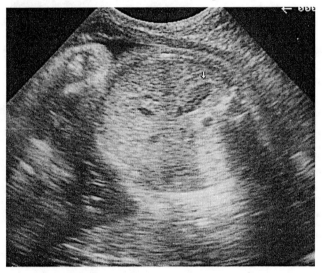

    A. Renal fossa
    B. Kidney
    C. Pelvis
    D. Adrenal gland
    E. Glisson's capsule

82. The bladder of the male fetus is sometimes enlarged because of:

    A. Imperforate hymen
    B. Posterior urethral valves
    C. Glands imperfecta
    D. Ureteropelvic junction
    E. Ectopic ureterocele

83. Ultrasonographically, fetal gender cannot be anatomically differentiated until:

    A. 10 weeks gestation
    B. 13 weeks gestation
    C. 16 weeks gestation
    D. 20 weeks gestation

E. 23 weeks gestation

84. The gender of this fetus is:

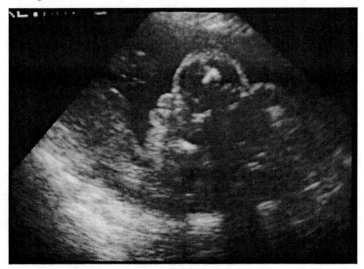

A. Male
B. Female
C. Ambiguous
D. XY
E. A and D

85. What structures can be seen routinely at the level of the bladder using a coronal view of the fetal pelvis on an obstetrical examination?

A. Shafts of the fetal fibula
B. Iliac bones
C. Sex characteristics
D. Knees
E. None of the above

86. When you have demonstrated the fetal stomach transversely at the level of the portal vein, you are at the appropriate level for:

A. Cord insertion
B. Thoracic circumference
C. Abdominal circumference
D. Fetal kidneys
E. Three-vessel cord

87. The obstetrical patient you are scanning complains of feeling dizzy, hot, and nauseated. This patient might be suffering from:

A. Hypertrophic cardiomyopathy
B. Hyperplasia
C. Hyperemesis gravederum
D. Hypertelorism

E. Supine hypotensive syndrome

88. A lab test that is performed to determine if a fetus has a neural tube defect or Down's syndrome is:

   A. MSAFP
   B. Triple screen
   C. CVS
   D. Amniocentesis
   E. All of the above

89. Which of the following lab tests can rule out Down's syndrome in at-risk patients?

   A. Ultrasound
   B. MSAFP
   C. Triple screen
   D. Amniocentesis
   E. Vesicocentesis

90. Second-trimester obstetrical ultrasound examinations are better than first-trimester sonograms in determining:

   A. Gestational age of the fetus
   B. Fetal birth weight
   C. Fetal position
   D. Fetal anatomy
   E. Fetal life

91. Characteristics of a biophysical profile include:

   A. Fetal breathing
   B. Fetal tone
   C. Fetal movement
   D. Amniotic fluid index
   E. All of the above

92. If you were observing the fetal forearm in the anatomical position, which of the following statements about the ulna would be TRUE?

   A. The ulna is longer than the radius proximally.
   B. The ulna is positioned lateral to the radius.
   C. The ulna and the radius end at the same level distally.
   D. A and B.
   E. A and C.

93. Which of the following statements about this image is NOT true?

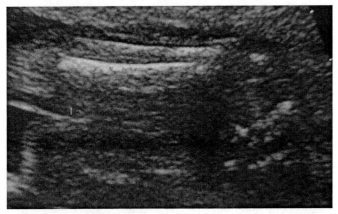

 A. It shows a good depiction of the sole of the foot.
 B. It shows a good foot position for measuring.
 C. It shows a good position for identifying club foot.
 D. All of the above.
 E. None of the above.

> **The following image applies to
> questions 94 and 95.**

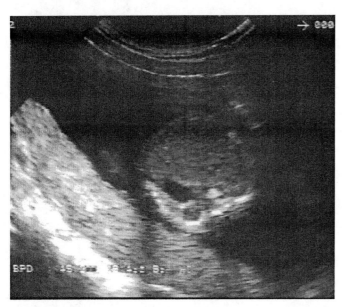

94. Judging from this transverse image of the maternal abdomen, what is the position of
the fetus?

 A. Transverse fetal head left
 B. Transverse fetal head right
 C. Vertex
 D. Breech
 E. Transverse spine up

95. If the previous image were taken longitudinally, the fetal lie would be:

    A. Transverse fetal head left
    B. Transverse fetal head right
    C. Vertex
    D. Breech
    E. Transverse spine up

96. While scanning an obstetrical patient, the first image that you have taken is a midline sagittal view of the lower uterine segment. If the cord is positioned near the cervical os, this is called:

    A. Partial previa
    B. Complete previa
    C. Vasa previa
    D. Cord presentation
    E. A and C

97. Physicians usually do not start to consider a Cesarean section due to placental previa until the:

    A. 25th week of gestation
    B. 30th week of gestation
    C. 37th week of gestation
    D. 21st week of gestation
    E. 31st week of gestation

98. What anatomic structure is NOT demonstrated in this image?

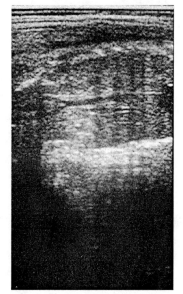

    A. Aortic bifurcation
    B. Right common iliac artery
    C. Left common iliac artery
    D. Ascending aorta

E. Descending aorta

99. This image is sometimes obtained to help demonstrate:

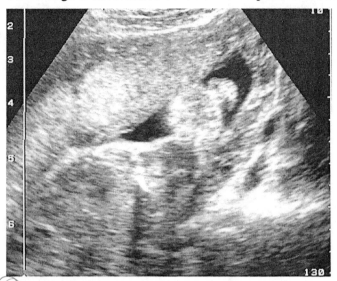

A. Cleft lip
B. Cleft palate
C. Encephalocele
D. B and C
E. A and C

100. To what is the arrow pointing in this longitudinal image through the fetal abdomen?

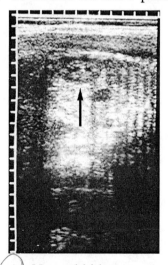

A. Normal kidney
B. Multicystic kidney
C. Polycystic kidney
D. Hydronephrotic kidney
E. Pseudo kidney mass

PLACENTA (1–5%)

Development

Position

Anatomy

Membranes

Umbilical cord

Abruption

Previa

Masses and lesions

Maturity/grading

Doppler

Physiology

Accreta

101. The placenta develops from the:

    A. Amnion
    B. Chorion
    C. Decidua
    D. A and B
    E. B and C

102. Umbilical cords can vary in length. A cord that appears to be abnormally thickened in an otherwise normal-appearing pregnancy is most likely the result of:

    A. Resistance of blood flow to the fetus
    B. Excessive Wharton's jelly
    C. Macrosomia
    D. Vascular duplication of the cord
    E. Cord edema

103. All of the following are functions of the placenta EXCEPT:

    A. Produces alphafetoprotein
    B. Secretes estrogen and progesterone
    C. Provides for diffusion of fetal wastes
    D. Serves as a source of nutrients
    E. Provides for an exchange of gasses

104. An accessory placental lobe is referred to as a(n) _____ placenta.

    A. Circumvallate
    B. Membranacea
    C. Succenturiate

D. Abruption

E. Battledore

105. A placenta previa can be ruled out if the placental edge is at least this distance from the internal cervical os.

A. 0.5 cm

B. 1 cm

C. 1.5 cm

D. 2 cm

E. 3 cm

106. In these two longitudinal scans through the lower uterine segment, one with full bladder and the other after partial voiding, what is the placental position?

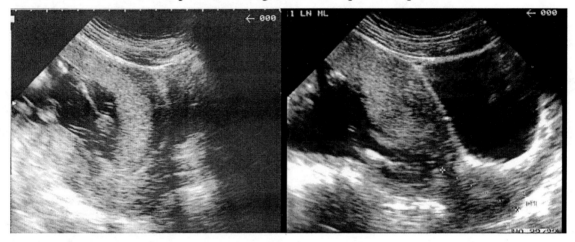

A. Anterior

B. Anterior previa

C. Anterior marginal

D. Anterior low lying

E. Total previa

107. One can rule out placenta accreta by observing:

A. Retroplacental space

B. Cord insertion

C. Placental texture

D. A and B

E. B and C

The image on the following page applies to questions 108 and 109.

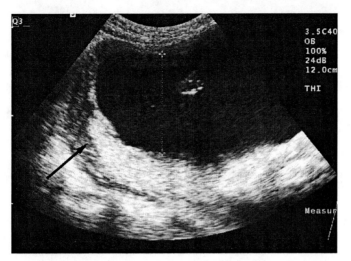

108. In this longitudinal scan through the uterus of an asymptomatic pregnant patient, the arrow is pointing to:

   A. An abruption
   B. Placental varicosities
   C. Myometrial contraction
   D. Cord insertion
   E. Normal retroplacental space

109. In the previous sonogram the position of the placenta:

   A. Anterior
   B. Posterior
   C. Fundal
   D. Lateral
   E. B and C

110. You are unable to identify the vascular space between placenta and myometrium. You suspect:

   A. Placenta accreta
   B. Abruption placenta
   C. Marginal placenta previa
   D. Succenturiate placenta
   E. Vasa previa

111. A placenta measuring 7 cm in greatest AP dimension may be associated with all of the following EXCEPT:

   A. Hydrops
   B. Infection
   C. Triploidy
   D. Hypertension
   E. Diabetes mellitus

112. The thickness of the full-term placenta should not measure more than:

    A. 2 cm
    B. 3 cm
    C. 4 cm
    D. 5 cm
    E. 6 cm

113. Which of the following statements about placental grading is <u>NOT</u> true?

    A. Placental grades range from 0–III.
    B. A grade III placenta indicates fetal lung maturity.
    C. Most placentas are grade II at delivery.
    D. Placental grading does not reliably predict fetal lung maturation.
    E. Diabetics often show a grade 0–I at term.

114. This structure was discovered during a routine obstetrical exam for gestational dating. It most likely represents:

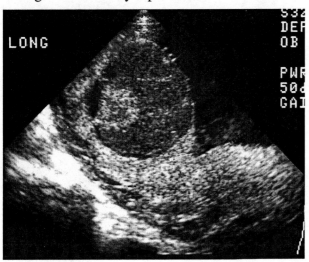

    A. Fibroid
    B. Myometrial contraction
    C. Abruption
    D. Chorioangioma
    E. Placental lake

115. The placenta in this image is grade:

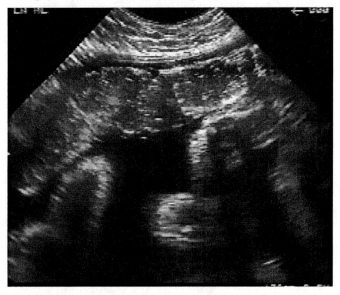

    A. 0
    B. I
    C. II
    D. III
    E. IV

116. To demonstrate the umbilical cord insertion into the fetal abdomen, one would look:

    A. Superior to the fetal kidneys
    B. Superior to the fetal bladder
    C. Posterior to the fetal stomach
    D. Posterior to the umbilical vein
    E. At the level of the adrenal glands

117. Refer to the two images on the following page to answer this question. The first image of an early second-trimester pregnancy and the second image with arrows pointing to the umbilical arteries on either side of the fetal bladder demonstrate:

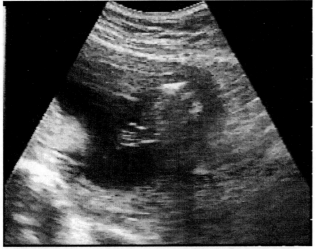

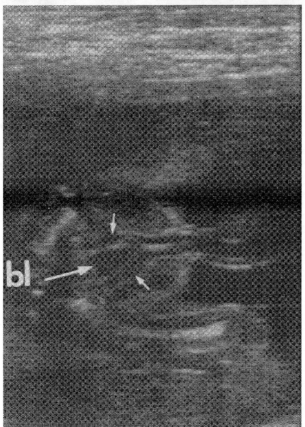

Reprinted with permission from Filly RA, Feldstein VA: Ultrasound evaluation of normal fetal anatomy. In Callen PW (ed): *Ultrasonography in Obstetrics and Gynecology*, 4th edition. Philadelphia, WB Saunders, 2000, p 251.

A. Three-vessel cord
B. Skin edema
C. Gastroschisis
D. Cord insertion
E. Omphalocele

118. Applying color Doppler to the transverse image through the fetal bladder will help verify:

    A. Normal femoral arteries
    B. Two umbilical arteries
    C. Single umbilical vein
    D. Aortic bifurcation
    E. Bladder function

119. A patient presents with severe abdominal pain and vaginal bleeding. This sonogram demonstrates:

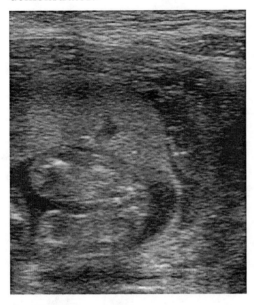

    A. Placenta previa
    B. Circumvallate placenta
    C. Placental abruption
    D. Marginal placenta
    E. Normal placenta

120. This patient presents with painless vaginal bleeding. The sonogram demonstrates:

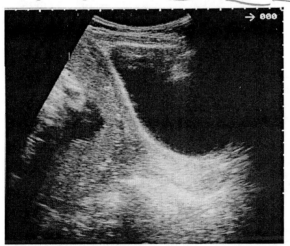

    A. Total placenta previa
    B. Circumvallate placenta

C. Anterior placental abruption

D. Posterior marginal placenta

E. Normal fundal placenta

ASSESSMENT OF GESTATIONAL AGE [2–6%]

Gestational sac

Embryonic size/crown-rump length

Biparietal diameter

Femur length

Abdominal circumference

Head circumference

Transcerebellar measurements

Binocular measurements

Cephalic indices

Fetal lung maturity

Other

///

121. The biparietal diameter and head circumference measurements are best taken at which level of the fetal brain?

   A. Falx cerebri
   B. Lateral ventricles
   C. Cerebral thalami
   D. Cerebellum
   E. Cisterna magna

122. Given an OFD of 70 mm and a BPD of 43 mm, calculate the cephalic index.

   A. 50%
   B. 61%
   C. 75%
   D. 80%
   E. 86%

123. The cephalic index in the previous question suggests:

   A. Dolichocephaly
   B. Brachycephaly
   C. Anencephaly
   D. Holoprosencephaly
   E. Ventriculomegaly

124. The best method and time for estimating gestational age would be:

A. Gestational sac measurement at 5 weeks
B. Crown-rump length at 10 weeks
C. Biparietal diameter at 15 weeks
D. Abdominal circumference at 20 weeks
E. Femur length at 30 weeks

125. Cerebellar measurements can be used to estimate gestational age but lose accuracy after:

    A. 15 weeks
    B. 20 weeks
    C. 25 weeks
    D. 30 weeks
    E. 35 weeks

126. Epiphyseal centers will not be identified sonographically until after:

    A. 20 weeks
    B. 25 weeks
    C. 30 weeks
    D. 35 weeks
    E. 40 weeks

127. Regarding BPD measurement, the practice of positioning the calipers on the outer edge of the anterior skull table and on the inner edge of the posterior skull table is termed:

    A. Cephalic index
    B. Leading edge
    C. Crucial parameter
    D. Peripheral dimension
    E. Biometric ratio

128. Fetal lung maturity is best determined by:

    A. Biometric evaluation
    B. Echogenicity of lungs
    C. Chorionic villus sampling
    D. Amniocentesis
    E. Alphafetoprotein levels

129. The cephalic index is performed to determine:

    A. Gestational age
    B. Mental capacity
    C. Head shape
    D. Fetal weight
    E. Lung maturity

130. One can calculate a patient's clinical due date by adding 9 months plus 7 days to the first day of the last menstrual period. This calculation is done according to:

    A. Naegele's rule
    B. McDonald's measurement
    C. Hadley's chart
    D. Old wives' tale
    E. Huygen's law

131. Of the following signs, which would NOT be present in the first trimester?

    A. Hegar's sign
    B. Chadwick's sign
    C. Quickening
    D. Sonographic fetal heart motion
    E. Amenorrhea

132. With normal growth during the first trimester, the size of the gestational sac should increase daily by:

    A. 1 mm
    B. 2 mm
    C. 5 mm
    D. 10 mm
    E. 1 cm

133. If no embryo is seen within a sac, one can roughly calculate the gestational age in weeks by measuring the mean sac diameter and adding ___ to it:

    A. 1
    B. 2
    C. 3
    D. 4
    E. 5

134. Sac measurements are accurate in estimating gestational age to within:

    A. 1 week
    B. 2 weeks
    C. 3 weeks
    D. 4 weeks
    E. 6 weeks

135. Which formula is used to calculate the cephalic index?

    A. (BPD + OFD) x 3.14
    B. (BPD + OFD) x 1.57
    C. (BPD + OFD) x 1.62
    D. BPD/OFD x 100
    E. (OFD – BPD) / 100

136. Which of the following measurements would NOT be used to confirm gestational age?

    A. Cerebellar length
    B. Binocular distance
    C. Renal length
    D. Humerus length
    E. Nuchal skin fold

137. Determining the tilt of the fetal head within the uterus is helpful in obtaining the correct angle for BPD and head circumference measurements. This is called finding the:

    A. Angle of asynclitism
    B. Presentation
    C. Corrected BPD
    D. Fetal lie
    E. Cephalic index

138. Which long bone is LEAST likely to be affected by intrauterine growth restriction?

    A. Femur
    B. Humerus
    C. Clavicle
    D. Tibia
    E. Radius

139. You are measuring abdominal circumference. You choose to do so at the level of the:

    A. Fetal kidneys
    B. Fetal stomach
    C. Cord insertion site
    D. Fetal gallbladder
    E. B and D

140. Which of the following statements about measuring the fetal head circumference would be considered TRUE?

    A. It is taken at the level of the lateral ventricles.
    B. It is considered more accurate than the biparietal diameter measurement.
    C. It is considered less accurate than the biparietal diameter measurement.
    D. A and B
    E. A and C

COMPLICATIONS [6–10%]

Intrauterine growth retardation (symmetrical, asymmetrical, nonstress test, biophysical
profile, Doppler flow studies)

Multiple gestations (diamniotic, monoamniotic, complications)

Maternal illness (gestational diabetes, diabetes mellitus, hypertension, other)

Antepartum (preterm labor, premature rupture of membranes, RH isoimmunization, cervix
related, other)

Fetal therapy (fetal blood sampling/transfusion, other)

Postpartum (hemorrhage, infection, caesarean section, other)

///

141. Which of the following best describes the function of the non-stress test?

    A. It calculates gestational age and fetal heart rate
    B. It calculates fetal heart rate according to fetal activity
    C. It calculates fetal heart rate according to uterine contractions
    D. It calculates fetal heart rate during fetal rest periods
    E. It calculates fetal heart and respiratory movements

142. All of the following are associated with nonimmune hydrops EXCEPT:

    A. Anasarca
    B. Pleural effusions
    C. Ascites
    D. Polyhydramnios
    E. Cleft defects

143. Twins resulting from the fertilization of a single ova are referred to as:

    A. Monozygotic
    B. Dizygotic
    C. Monoamniotic
    D. Dichorionic
    E. Fraternal

144. Which of these statements about twins is NOT true?

    A. 100% of dizygotic twins are dichorionic.
    B. Monozygotic twins share the same amniotic sac.
    C. Twin-to-twin transfusion syndrome is specific to monozygotic gestations.
    D. Monozygotic twins can be dichorionic.
    E. Chorionicity is related to placentation.

145. Which of the following anomalies is associated specifically with maternal diabetes mellitus?

    A. Turner's syndrome
    B. Potter's syndrome
    C. Thanatophoric dwarfism
    D. Caudal regression syndrome
    E. Osteogenesis imperfecta

146. If a patient's AFP level is low, one should check for:

    A. Neural tube defects
    B. Multiple gestation
    C. Abdominal wall defects
    D. Trisomy 21
    E. Skeletal dysplasia

147. Which statement about fetal brain anatomy is TRUE?

    A. Ventricular measurements are consistent throughout pregnancy.
    B. BPD and head circumference measurements are taken at the level of the cerebellum.
    C. The choroid plexus sits within the anterior horn of the lateral ventricle.
    D. Cerebral peduncles are at the level of the ventricles
    E. The cavum septum pellucidi are seen in the posterior fossa.

148. A skull that is shaped like a clover leaf is most likely to be associated with:

    A. Osteogenesis imperfecta
    B. Thanatophoric dwarfism
    C. Spina bifida aperta
    D. Sirenomelia
    E. Holoprosencephaly

149. You discover a rounded, fluid-filled midline structure within the fetal brain. When color Doppler is employed, the structure shows color. The most likely diagnosis would be:

    A. Choroid plexus cyst
    B. Arachnoid cyst
    C. Dilation of the 3rd ventricle
    D. Vein of Galen aneurysm
    E. Dandy-Walker malformation

150. All of the following statements about alobar holoprosencephaly are true EXCEPT:

    A. It is compatible with life and carries a good prognosis
    B. It is associated with cleft defects of the face.
    C. It is associated with Trisomy 13.
    D. There is a large monoventricle with fused thalami.
    E. It is usually fatal.

151. If a patient's menstrual dates are not known, which ratio is most sensitive for detecting asymmetrical intrauterine growth restriction?

    A. HC/AC
    B. Cephalic index
    C. FL/AC
    D. BPD/AC
    E. Amniotic fluid index

152. Which of the following would not be associated with oligohydramnios? DRIPP

    A. Intrauterine growth restriction
    B. Premature rupture of membranes
    C. Bilateral renal agenesis
    D. Intrauterine fetal demise
    E. GI tract obstruction

153. The obstetrical patient who presents with hypertension, swelling, and proteinuria is said to have:

    A. Preeclampsia
    B. Toxemia
    C. Eclampsia
    D. A and B
    E. B and C

154. Which cardiac abnormality cannot be detected with the four-chamber view?

    A. Transposition of the great vessels
    B. Hypoplastic left ventricle
    C. Ventricular septal defect
    D. Complete heart block
    E. Cardiomegaly

155. The basic guidelines for obstetrical scanning require us to take four fetal measurements. Which of the following is NOT one of those measurements?

    A. BPD
    B. Head circumference
    C. Ventricular diameter
    D. Abdominal circumference
    E. Femur length

156. When the fetus is breech or cephalic and one scans the maternal abdomen in the sagittal plane, the tilt of the fetal head in the uterus can be assessed. By scanning perpendicular to the tilt of the fetal head, one can obtain the proper level for measuring the fetal head. This is called the angle of:

    A. Cerclage
    B. Asynclitism

C. McDonald
D. Biparietalism
E. Occiput

157. This image leads you to suspect:

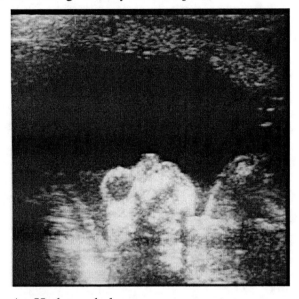

A. Hydrocephalus
B. Anencephaly
C. Acrania
D. Encephalocele
E. Cleft palate

158. Refer to the following two images for this question. In these longitudinal images of the frontal view of the fetal face, the arrows point to:

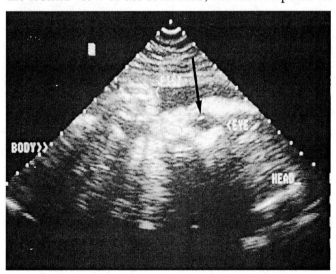

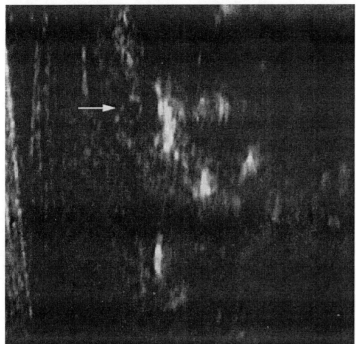

Reprinted with permission from Babcook CJ: The fetal face and neck. In Callen PW (ed): *Ultrasonography in Obstetrics and Gynecology*, 4th edition. Philadelphia, WB Saunders, 2000, p 310.

A. Upper lip
B. Nasal bones
C. Lens of the eye
D. Proboscis
E. Tongue

159. This longitudinal image on the following page of the fetal thorax demonstrates:

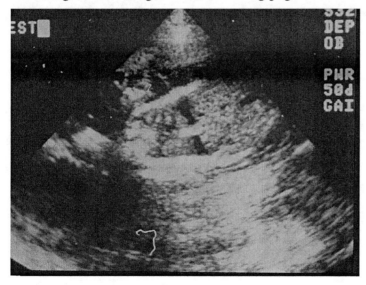

A. Abdominal ascites
B. Anasarca
C. Pericardial fluid
D. Pleural effusions
E. Normal thorax

160. This transverse image taken through the fetal neck demonstrates:

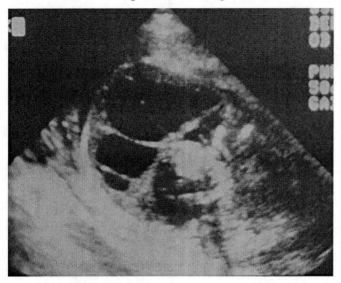

    A. Pleural effusions
    B. Anasarca
    C. Teratoma
    D. Cystic hygroma
    E. Polyhydramnios

161. This finding is associated with which syndrome?

    A. Turner's
    B. Down's
    C. Potter's
    D. Fetal alcohol
    E. Caudal regression

162. A patient presents large for gestational age at 7–8 weeks LMP. This transverse image demonstrates:

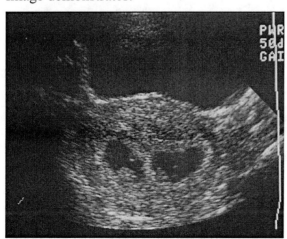

    A. Single sac with implantation bleed

    B. Polyhydramnios

    C. Split image artifact

    D. Twins

    E. Bicornuate uterus

163. Which of these tests is best for determining fetal lung maturity?

    A. Chorionic villus sampling

    B. Lecithin/sphingomyelin ratio

    C. BPD/FL ratio

    D. Placental grading

    E. Fetal lung tissue characterization

164. The term *puerperium* refers to which period?

    A. Before delivery

    B. First trimester

    C. Second trimester

    D. Third trimester

    E. After delivery

165. The postpartum uterus should revert back to pregravid size within:

    A. 72 hours

    B. 1 week

    C. 2 weeks

    D. 3 weeks

    E. 4 weeks

166. A molar pregnancy associated with a viable fetus is called a:

    A. Hydatidiform mole

    B. Chorioadenoma destruens

    C. Choriocarcinoma

    D. Coexistent mole and live fetus

    E. Breus' mole

167. On physical exam, all of the following would cause a patient to present large for gestational age EXCEPT:

    A. Cystadenoma

    B. Cystic teratoma

    C. Myometrial contraction

    D. Leiomyomas

    E. Trophoblastic disease

168. In this sonogram of a second-trimester pregnancy the arrow is pointing to:

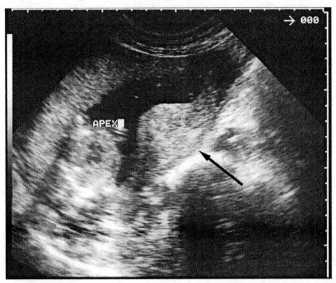

    A. A leiomyoma
    B. A chorioangioma
    C. The placenta
    D. The fetal trunk
    E. A contraction

169. Which statement is NOT true of dizygotic twinning?

    A. It is more common among African Americans than Caucasians.
    B. There is an increased incidence if the father was a twin.
    C. Women over 40 have a higher incidence.
    D. Dizygotic twins are considered fraternal twins.
    E. Dizygotic twinning is more common than monozygotic twinning in the US.

170. Twin growth is similar to that of singletons up to:

    A. 10 weeks
    B. 15 weeks
    C. 20 weeks
    D. 25 weeks
    E. 30 weeks

171. All of the following are associated specifically with monozygotic twins EXCEPT:

    A. Twin-to-twin transfusion syndrome
    B. TRAP sequence
    C. Conjoined twins
    D. Erythroblastosis fetalis
    E. Cord entanglement

172. Maternal hypertension would NOT be associated with:

    A. Macrosomia

B. IUGR
C. Advanced placental grade for age
D. Fetal demise
E. Oligohydramnios

173. Which drug is given to the RH– mother to protect against alloimmunization?

A. Pergonal
B. Rhogam
C. Methotrexate
D. Indomethacin
E. Tetracycline

174. Which of these statements about intrauterine fetal blood transfusion is TRUE?

A. It cannot be performed prenatally.
B. Packed red blood cells are introduced into the umbilical arteries.
C. Packed red blood cells are introduced into the umbilical vein.
D. The puncture should be made as the cord enters the fetal abdomen.
E. Cordocentesis is most successfully performed when the placenta is lateral.

175. The most common surgical procedure during pregnancy is:

A. Cerclage procedure
B. Cesarean section
C. Wedge resection
D. Salpingoophorectomy
E. Appendectomy

176. Which of the following statements is NOT true?

A. Pregnancy may be a cause for the development of gallstones.
B. Hormonal changes of pregnancy increase the likelihood of venous thrombosis.
C. Pelvicaliectasis, during pregnancy, is most often observed on the left side.
D. During the third trimester, an inflamed appendix would be observed more cephalic in location.
E. During pregnancy, tenderness over the kidneys should suggest pyelonephritis.

177. A molar pregnancy that is considered invasive but does not metastasize is called:

A. Choriocarcinoma
B. Chorioadenoma destruens
C. Hydatidiform mole
D. Partial mole
E. Pseudo mole

178. A habitual aborter has undergone a McDonald's procedure. To what is the arrow pointing in this longitudinal scan through the lower uterine segment?

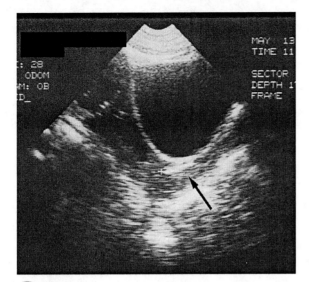

A. Cerclage
B. Tampon
C. Scar
D. Calcification
E. IUD

179. A McDonald's procedure is performed to:

    A. Remove an IUD
    B. Freeze the cervix for dysplasia
    C. Treat an incompetent cervix
    D. Treatment to enhance fertility
    E. Artificially inseminate

180. The postpartum periods lasts:

    A. 2–4 weeks
    B. 6–8 weeks
    C. 10–12 weeks
    D. 12–14 weeks
    E. 1 month

181. The most common cause of acute postpartum hemorrhage is:

    A. Retained products of conception
    B. Succenturiate placenta
    C. Endometritis
    D. Uterine atony
    E. Uterine fibroids

182. Twin reversed arterial perfusion (TRAP) results in:

    A. Twin-to-twin transfusion
    B. Acardiac twin
    C. Conjoined twins

D. Fraternal twins

E. Vanishing twin

183. A fetus that weighs 4600 grams at term is said to be:

    A. Macrosomic   *big baby*
    B. Growth-restricted
    C. Diabetic
    D. Post-term
    E. Small for gestational age (SGA)

184. Which of the following would NOT be likely to cause postpartum hemorrhage?

    A. Multiple gestation
    B. Polyhydramnios
    C. Macrosomia
    D. Long labor
    E. TORCH

185. Treatment for the pre-eclamptic patient includes all of the following EXCEPT:

    A. Hospitalization
    B. Bed rest
    C. Fetal biophysical profiles
    D. Diuretics
    E. Contraction stress tests

186. All of the following parameters are evaluated in the fetal biophysical profile EXCEPT:

    A. Fetal tone
    B. Fetal breathing
    C. Fetal eye movement
    D. Fetal body movement
    E. Amniotic fluid

187. Of the following conditions, which is NOT associated with a thick, edematous placenta?

    A. Maternal diabetes
    B. Erythroblastosis fetalis
    C. TORCH
    D. Non-immune hydrops
    E. Pregnancy induced hypertension

AMNIOTIC FLUID [1–5%]

Assessment

Polyhydramnios

Oligohydramnios

Fetal pulmonic maturity studies

188. Of the following amniotic fluid indices, which would be considered polyhydramnios?

    A. 3 cm
    B. 9 cm
    C. 15 cm
    — D. 24 cm
    E. None of the above

189. Which of the following is least likely to be associated with polyhydramnios?

    A. Neural tube defect
    — B. Intrauterine growth restriction
    C. Omphalocele
    D. Dwarfism
    E. Twins

190. Which of the following would NOT be considered a function of amniotic fluid?

    A. Allows for normal development of musculoskeletal system
    B. Regulates body heat
    C. Provides a means of protection
    D. Allows for normal lung development
    — E. Provides nourishment

191. The quantitative method of determining whether the amniotic fluid level is normal or not is called:

    — A. Amniotic fluid index
    B. Eyeballing
    C. Qualitative evaluation
    D. Amniocentesis
    E. Uterine volume

192. Green-tinged particles floating in amniotic fluid most likely are:

    A. Spinach that Mom ate for lunch
    B. Vernix
    — C. Meconium
    D. Shed skin
    E. Shed hair

193. Amniotic fluid is produced by the:

     A. Fetal liver
     B. Fetal gut
     C. Fetal kidneys
     D. Placenta
     E. Choroids plexus

GENETIC STUDIES [1–3%]

Maternal serum testing

Amniotic fluid testing

Chorionic villus sampling

Dominate/recessive risk occurrence

194. MSAFP results are reported in the following unit of measurement:

     A. Lectin/sphingomyelin (L/S)
     B. Positive predictive value (PPV)
     C. Multiples of the median (MoM)
     D. Phosphatidyl glycerol (PG)
     E. Acetylcholinesterase (ACHE)

195. A triple marker screening (triple test) measures:

     A. Unconjugated estriol (uE3)
     B. Acetyl cholinesterase (ACHE)
     C. Human chorionic gonadotropin (hCG)
     D. Alpha-fetoprotein (AFP)
     E. A, C, and D

196. Which of the following is not associated with an elevated MSAFP?

     A. Abdominal wall defects
     B. Fetal demise
     C. Hydatidiform mole
     D. Maternal renal abnormalities
     E. Multiple gestation

197. Which of the following is NOT associated with a decreased MSAFP?

     A. Death of the fetus
     B. Underestimation of gestational age
     C. Missed abortion
     D. Gastrointestinal obstruction
     E. Hydatidiform mole

198. Acetyl cholinesterase (ACHE) is most specific for which of the following?

    —A. Spina bifida
    B. Down's syndrome
    C. Trisomy 13
    D. Trisomy 18
    E. Triploidy

199. Which of the following statements about Down's syndrome is FALSE?

    A. Enlarged nuchal thickness in some cases
    B. Abnormal triple screen
    C. Decreased MSAFP
    —D. Amniocentesis sometimes unnecessary for prenatal diagnosis
    E. Increased incidence with increased maternal age

200. Which of the following is/are standardly used to determine fetal lung maturity?

    A. L/S (lecithin/sphingomyelin)and PG (phosphatidylglycerol)
    B. ACHE (acetyl cholinesterase)
    C. Amniocentesis
    D. A and B
    —E. A and C

201. The risk of complications is highest for:

    A. Amniocentesis
    B. CVS (chorionic villus sampling)
    —C. PUBS (percutaneous umbilical blood sampling)
    D. A and B
    E. B and C

202. For best results, the optimal gestational age for karyotyping by amniocentesis is:

    A. 12–13 weeks
    —B. 15–16 weeks
    C. 18–20 weeks
    D. 22–24 weeks
    E. 26–28 weeks

203. Which of the following is NOT true about chorionic villus sampling (CVS):

    A. The sample is taken from the chorion frondosum.
    B. CVS provides a means of early diagnosis.
    C. The waiting period for results is shorter than that for other tests.
    D. Spotting is common following the procedure.
    — E. The transabdominal technique is most commonly used.

204. At what gestational age are chorionic villus sampling procedures commonly performed?

A. 5–7 weeks
B. 7–9 weeks
C. 10–13 weeks
D. 15–16 weeks
E. 17–18 weeks

205. A disorder that is caused by the presence of only one defective gene is called:

A. Autosomal recessive
B. Autosomal dominant
C. X-linked
D. A and C
E. All of the above

206. Which of the following statements is TRUE for an x-linked disease:

A. The mother must have the disease in order to pass it on to her children.
B. The father must have the disease in order to pass it on to his children.
C. It is an autosomal dominant disorder.
D. 100% of all female offspring will have the disease process.
E. None of the above

FETAL DEMISE [0–3%]

207. Which of the following statements is NOT true about fetal demise:

A. Absence of cardiac motion for at least 3 minutes is a sonographic hallmark.
B. The diagnosis should be confirmed by more than one examiner.
C. Failure of mother to feel fetal movement is diagnostic
D. Spalding's sign might be present.
E. Deuel's sign might be present.

208. What is *lithopedion*?

A. Calcium deficiency
B. Fetal gallstones
C. Calcified fetus
D. Lack of fetal tone
E. Fusion of bone

209. The most common cause of fetal death in the third trimester is:

A. Maternal uterine anomalies
B. Intrauterine infections
C. Maternal diabetes mellitus
D. Chromosomal abnormalities
E. Unknown cause

210. This transverse image demonstrates:

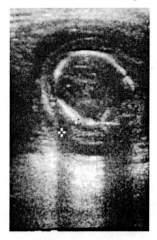

    A. The banana sign
    B. The lemon sign
    C. Spaulding's sign
— D. Deuel's sign (halo sign)
    E. None of the above

211. The most common cause of fetal demise in the first trimester is:

    A. Maternal uterine anomalies
    B. Intrauterine infections
    C. Maternal diabetes mellitus
— D. Chromosomal abnormalities
    E. Unknown cause

212. The following condition is an indication for immediate delivery, for without it there is the risk of intrauterine demise:

    A. Vasa previa
— B. Placental abruption
    C. Incompetent cervix
    D. Uterine infection
    E. Implantation bleed

213. Which of the following is/are common medical intervention(s) for the removal of retained products of conception (RPOC)?

    A. Dilatation and curettage
    B. Dilation and evacuation
    C. Labor induction
    D. A and C only
— E. All of the above

214. A 30-year-old is 1 week postpartum and extremely anemic, exhausted, and just wants to sleep all of the time. You suspect:

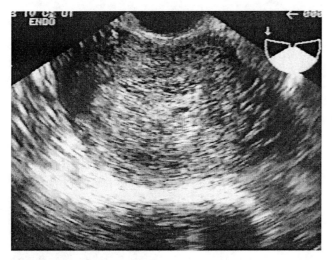

A. Endometrial cancer
B. Molar pregnancy
C. Fibroid uterus
— D. Retained products of conception (RPOC)
E. Uterine rupture

215. Which of the following is NOT likely to result from retained products of conception?

A. 2 weeks postpartum with heavy bleeding
B. Complex homogenous mass within endometrium with a + urine choriogonadotropin (UCG)
C. Echogenic mass in the cervix with a + UCG
— D. Pseudosac within endometrium with a + UCG
E. Acoustic shadowing from bony structures within uterine cavity.

216. The following image demonstrates:

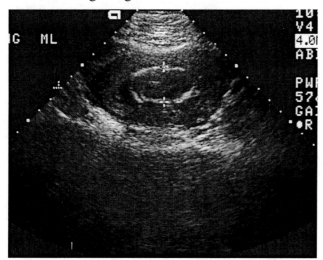

A. The banana sign
B. The lemon sign
— C. Spaulding's sign

D. Deuel's sign
E. None of the above

This image applies to questions 217–219.

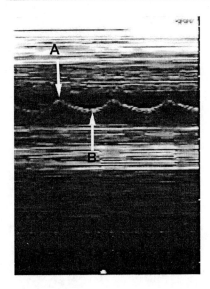

217. This image represents which of the following?

    A. A-mode
    B. B-mode
    C. D-mode
  — D. M-mode
    E. PW-mode

218. In the previous image, arrow *A* represents:

    A. Arrhythmia
  — B. Systole
    C. Diastole
    D. Aliasing
    E. None of the above

219. Arrow *B* in the same image represents:

    A. Arrhythmia
    B. Systole
  — C. Diastole
    D. Aliasing
    E. None of the above

FETAL ABNORMALITIES [10–15%]

Cranial

Facial

Neck

Neural tube

Abdominal wall

Thoracic

Genitourinary

Gastrointestinal

Skeletal

Cardiac

Syndromes

Other

/ /

220. Which of the following is not associated with holoprosencephaly?

    A. Failed development of the fetal forebrain
    — B. Failure of the cranial vault to form correctly
    C. Proboscis
    D. Cyclopia
    E. Fused thalami

221. The most common neural tube defect is:

    A. Spina bifida aperta
    — B. Anencephaly
    C. Encephalocele
    D. Scoliosis
    E. Spina bifida occulta

222. Encephaloceles are usually found in the:

    — A. Occipital region
    B. Frontal regions
    C. Parietal regions
    D. A and B
    E. All of the above

223. Dangling or drooping choroid plexus is associated with:

    A. Porencephaly
    — B. Hydrocephalus

    C. Holoprosencephaly
    D. Dandy-Walker malformation
    E. Macrosomia

224. Which of the following can mimic anencephaly?

    A. Cystic hygroma
    B. Rhombencephalon
 ── C. Microcephaly
    D. Encephalocele
    E. Dandy-Walker malformation

225. Which of the following is the result of a defect in the cranium and herniation of cranial meninges through the defect?

 ── A. Encephalocele
    B. Daryocystoceles
    C. Cystic hygroma
    D. Holoprosencephaly
    E. Anencephaly

226. Which of the following are not associated with Dandy-Walker malformation?

    A. Hydrocephalus
    B. Posterior fossa cyst
 ── C. Arises from the cerebrum
    D. Agenesis of the corpus callosum
    E. Enlarged 4th ventricle

227. The arrow in the image is pointing to:

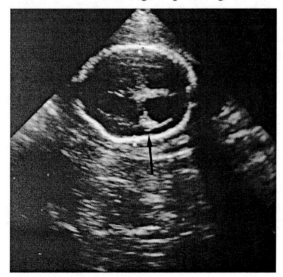

    A. Choroid plexus cyst
    B. Deuel's sign
 ── C. Dangling choroid
    D. Spalding sign

E. None of the above

228. What would cause this to happen?

A. Infarction
B. Fetal death
— C. Hydrocephalus
D. Anencephaly
E. All of the above

229. Holoprosencephaly is most often associated with which of the following?

— A. Trisomy 13
B. Trisomy 18
C. Trisomy 21
D. Triploidy
E. Down's syndrome

230. Which of the following is or are TRUE about macrosomia?

A. It frequently is associated with the diabetic patient.
B. The fetal body is smaller than the abdomen.
C. The fetal head and abdomen are enlarged.
D. A and B
— E. A and C

231. What anomaly would you expect to be associated with this finding?

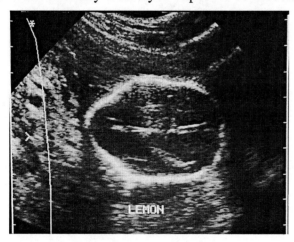

A. Dwarfism
B. Down's syndrome
— C. Spina bifida
D. Macrosomia
E. Anasarca

232. What else might you expect to see with this anomaly?

A. Large head circumference

B. Flattened cerebellum
C. Shortened femur
D. Hydrops
E. Protruding forehead

233. A cyst within the fetal brain that is thought almost always to regress with fetal age is:

   A. Dandy-Walker cyst
   B. Cystic hygroma
   C. Encephalocele
   —D. Choroid plexus cyst
   E. None of the above

234. The following image demonstrates:

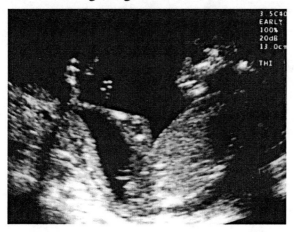

   A. Micrognathia
   B. Clubfoot
   C. Encephalocele
   — D. Anencephaly
   E. Microcephaly

235. Which of the following is TRUE about hydranencephaly?

   A. Poor prognosis
   B. Complete destruction of the cerebrum
   C. Bilateral clefts in the cerebrum
   — D. A and B
   E. A and C

236. Facial abnormalities can be associated with chromosomal abnormalities. Which of the following is not commonly detected by ultrasound?

   A. Cleft lip
   —B. Low-set ears
   C. Cyclopia
   D. Micrognathia

E. Hypertelorism

237. The findings in this image of the fetal head strongly suggest:

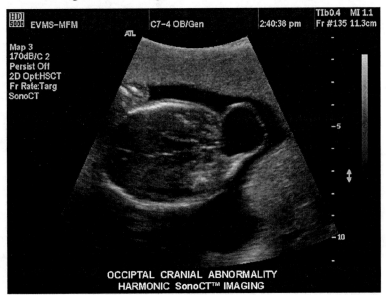

A. Encephalocele
B. Hydrocephalus
C. Trisomy 13
D. Down syndrome
E. Fetal demise

238. The following image of the fetal profile suggests:

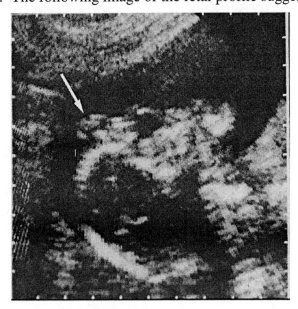

A. Normal profile
B. Absence of the nasal bridge
C. Micrognathia
D. Protuberant forehead
E. Hypertelorism

239. When the condition in the image from the previous question and proboscis are seen together, you would first suspect:

    A. Trisomy 21
    B. Trisomy 18
    C. Triploidy
    — D. Cyclopia
    E. Schizencephaly

240. Hypotelorism is associated with:

    A. Normal pregnancy
    B. Wide-spaced eyes
    — C. Cyclopia
    D. IUGR
    E. Down syndrome

241. Which is the best description of micrognathia?

    A. Moderate posterior position of the frontal bone
    — B. Moderate posterior position of the mandible
    C. Decrease in the normal size of the nasal bone
    D. Decrease in the normal size of the tongue
    E. Absence of the nasal septum

242. Cystic hygromas are often associated with which of the following?

    A. Potter's type II
    — B. Turner's syndrome
    C. Prune belly syndrome
    D. Dandy-Walker malformation
    E. Arnold-Chiari malformation

243. Of the following choices, what would be the most likely diagnosis from this image?

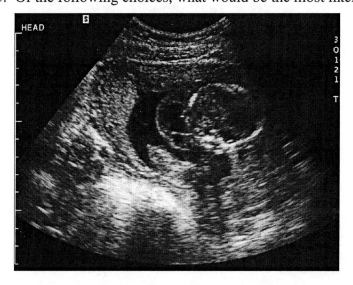

   A. Encephalocele
   B. Spina bifida
 — C. Cystic hygroma
   D. Down's syndrome
   E. Nuchal translucency

244. At what gestational age is nuchal fold thickness usually measured?

   A. 10–14 weeks
 — B. 15–21 weeks
   C. 22–24 weeks
   D. 25–28 weeks
   E. 29–32 weeks

245. The most common abnormality associated with the central nervous system is:

   A. Encephalocele
   B. Hydrocephalus
 — C. Anencephaly
   D. Spina bifida occulta
   E. Holoprosencephaly

246. The arrows in this image demonstrate:

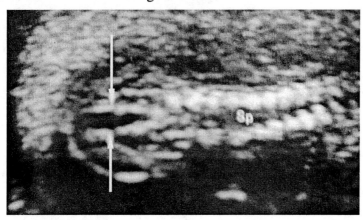

   A. Hemivertebra
 — B. Spina bifida
   C. Spondylolisthesis
   D. Rachischisis
   E. Scoliosis

247. A spinal defect containing meninges and neural tissue is called a/an:

   A. Encephalocele
   B. Spina bifida
   C. Meningocele
 — D. Meningomyelocele
   E. Omphalocele

248. What are the arrows pointing to in this image?

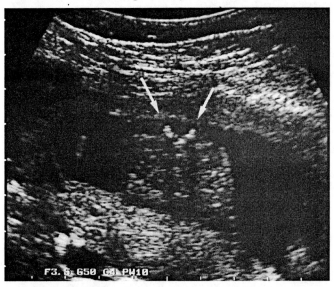

   A. Splaying of the transverse processes
 — B. Splaying of the laminae
   C. Spalding's sign
   D. Anasarca
   E. None of the above

249. A sonographer can BEST distinguish between a gastroschisis and an omphalocele by visualizing the:

 — A. Cord insertion
   B. The contents of the mass
   C. A membrane
   D. Kidneys
   E. 3-vessel cord

250. To what is the arrow pointing in this image?

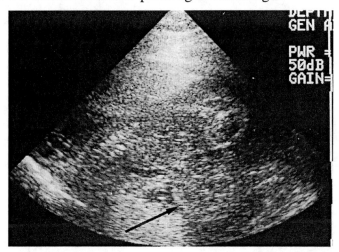

   A. Conjoined twins
   B. Gastroschisis

   —C. Omphalocele
   D. Hiatal hernia
   E. Spina bifida

251. Which of the following statements is NOT true of gastroschisis?

   A. There is a normal cord insertion
   — B. It is covered by peritoneum
   C. It is associated with preterm delivery
   D. It is not associated with other anomalies
   E. Sometimes difficult to see using ultrasound

252. Of the following anomalies involving abdominal wall defects, which is usually
   NOT compatible with life?

   A. Omphalocele
   B. Gastroschisis
   C. Bladder exstrophy
   D. Cloacal exstrophy
   — E. Limb/body wall complex

253. This image best demonstrates:

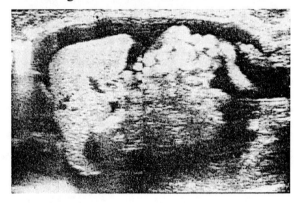

   A. Gastroschisis
   B. Pleural effusion
   C. Fetal demise
   — D. Fetal ascites
   E. None of the above

254. Transabdominal ultrasound reveals a soft-tissue mass protruding from the anterior
   wall of the fetus just inferior to the cord insertion. The diagnostic possibilities
   include:

   A. Bladder exstrophy
   B. Cloacal exstrophy
   C. Gastrointestinal teratoma
   — D. A and B
   E. All of the above

255. Which of the following is NOT associated with fetal hydrops?

    A. Pleural effusion
    B. Anasarca
— C. Megacystis
    D. Ascites
    E. Pericardial effusion

256. Which statement is NOT characteristic of congenital cystic adenomatoid malformation (CCAM)?

    A. Can become very large
— B. Can be determined only by biopsy
    C. Associated with fetal hydrops
    D. Polyhydramnios often identified
    E. Can be solid in appearance

257. Sonography demonstrates a localized cystic-appearing structure adjacent to the fetal heart that displaces the heart along the anterior chest wall. These findings most likely represent:

    A. Pleural effusion
    B. Pericardial effusion
    C. Lung sequestration
— D. Diaphragmatic hernia
    E. Pulmonary atresia

258. This image reveals a(n):

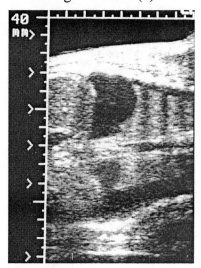

    A. Anasarca
    B. Abdominal ascites
— C. Pleural effusion
    D. Thickened diaphragm
    E. Pneumothorax

259. A congenital diaphragmatic hernia can be associated with all of the following EXCEPT:

    A. Abnormal shift of the fetal heart
    B. Compression of the fetal lungs
— C. Pulmonary hyperplasia
    D. Failure of the diaphragm to form properly
    E. Neural tube defects

260. The most common renal abnormality in an unborn fetus is:

    A. Multicystic kidney
    B. Polycystic kidney
— C. Hydronephrosis
    D. Potter's syndrome Type I
    E. Potter's syndrome Type II

261. What is being measured in this transverse image through the region of the fetal kidneys?

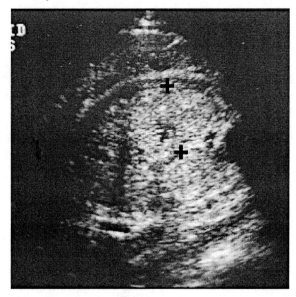

    A. Normal right kidney
— B. Polycystic kidney
    C. Multicystic kidney
    D. Dilated renal pelvis
    E. Mass of unknown etiology

262. If one identifies a dilated bladder, megaureters, and hydronephrosis, one should suspect:

    A. Stone
    B. Imperforate hymen
— C. Posterior urethral valves (PUV) obstruction
    D. Ureteropelvic junction obstruction (UPJ)
    E. Ureterovesical junction obstruction (UVJ)

263. The most likely cause of unilateral hydronephrosis is:

    A. Posterior urethral valve obstruction
    B. Multicystic kidney disease
    C. Wilm's tumor
    D. Ureteropelvic junction obstruction
    E. Prune Belly syndrome

264. Which of the following is NOT associated with oligohydramnios?

    A. PROM
    B. Intrauterine growth restriction (IUGR)
    C. Posterior urethral valves obstruction (PUV)
    D. Unilateral ureteropelvic junction (UPJ) obstruction
    E. Potter's Type I

265. The congenital absence of the kidneys bilaterally and severe oligohydramnios suggest:

    A. Classic Potter's syndrome
    B. Potter's syndrome Type I
    C. Potter's syndrome Type II
    D. Potter's syndrome Type III
    E. Potter's syndrome Type IV

266. If arrow *B* is pointing to the bladder, arrow *A* is most likely pointing to the following structure superior to the bladder:

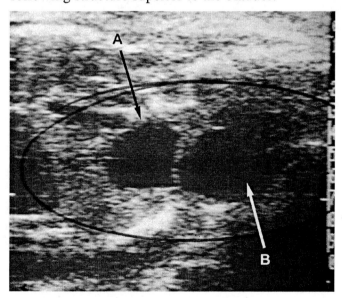

    A. Double bubble
    B. Urachal cyst
    C. Omphalocele
    D. Megacystis
    E. Torsion

267. What condition does this sonogram reveal posterior to the fetal stomach?

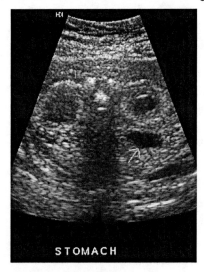

A. Bilateral pleural effusion
B. Hydronephrosis
C. Abdominal ascites
D. Dilated bowel loops
E. Urachal cyst

268. Visualization of the fetal heart and stomach in their correct positions rules out:

A. Esophageal atresia
B. Congenital diaphragmatic hernia
C. Situs inversus
D. A and C
E. All of the above

269. This image of the upper abdomen is an example of:

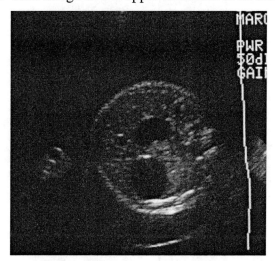

A. Double bubble
B. Duodenal atresia

    C. Bilateral hydronephrosis

— D. A and B

    E. Normal stomach

270. Echogenic bowel is usually associated with:

    A. Classic Potter's syndrome

    B. Fetal alcohol syndrome

    C. Turner's syndrome

→ D. Down's syndrome

    E. Trisomy 18

271. The term *double bubble* denotes:

    A. Fetal stomach next to heart

— B. Dilated duodenum next to the fetal stomach

    C. Bilateral hydronephrosis

    D. Choledochal cyst next to stomach

    E. Urachal cyst next to bladder

272. Bowing of the femur can be a result of:

    A. Hypophophatasia

    B. Artifact

    C. Sirenomielia or artifact

— D. Artifact or dysplasia

    E. Achondrogenesis, artifact, or dysplasia

273. Fracture of the femur can be a result of:

    A. Osteogenesis imperfecta

    B. Artifact

— C. Osteogenesis imperfecta and artifact

    D. Artifact and dysplasia

    E. Osteogenesis imperfecta, artifact, and dysplasia

274. What is *talipes*?

    A. Polydactyly

— B. Clubfoot

    C. Cleft lip

    D. Rocker bottom

    E. None of the above

275. Caudal regression syndrome is associated with:

    A. Diabetes

    B. Mermaid sign

    C. Sirenomelia

    D. B and C

— E. All of the above

276. Which of the following head shapes are associated with thanatophoric dysplasia?

    A. Strawberry
    B. Lemon
    C. Cloverleaf
    D. Brachycephaly
    E. Frontal bossing

277. Clinodactyly refers to:

    A. Wide-spaced digits
    B. Absence of digits
    C. Increased number of digits
    D. Permanent curvature or overlapping digits
    E. Fusion of the digits

278. Sirenomelia is associated with: *Mermaid syndrome – fused together*

    A. Deuel's sign
    B. Diabetic mothers
    C. Fusion of the lower limbs
    D. A and B
    E. B and C

279. This image demonstrates:

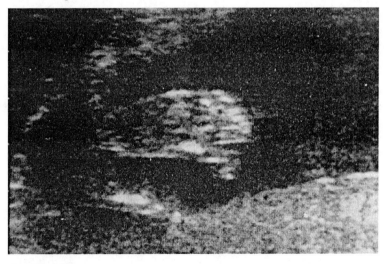

    A. Club foot
    B. Talipes
    C. Rocker bottom
    D. Polydactyly
    E. Sandal gap deformity

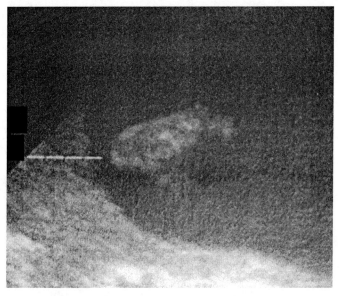

    A. Club foot
    B. Talipes
—   C. Rocker bottom
    D. Polydactyly
    E. Sandal foot

281. Double right outlet is almost always associated with:

    A. Pulmonary atresia
    B. Aortic stenosis
—   C. Hypoplastic left ventricle
    D. Arrhythmia
    E. Premature ventricular contractions (PVC)

282. Sonographic visualization of a cystic fluid-filled collection adjacent and posterior to the heart most likely represents:

    A. Cystic adenomatoid malformation
—   B. Congenital diaphragmatic hernia
    C. Pleural effusion
    D. Cardiac cyst
    E. Aortic aneurysm

283. Which of these congenital cardiac abnormalities cannot be diagnosed with the four-chamber view?

    A. Hypoplastic left ventricle
    B. Ventricular septal defect
—   C. Transposition of the great vessels
    D. Av block
    E. Pulmonary atresia

284. In this image the arrows point to:

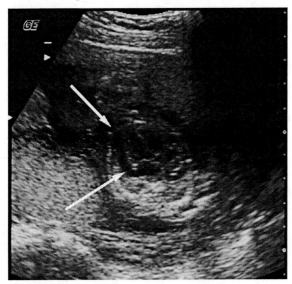

    A. Cardial myopathy
    B. Congestive heart failure
    C. Pleural effusion
   — D. Pericardial effusion
    E. Fetal ascites

285. Premature atrial contractions:

  — A. Are common and benign
    B. Always require treatment
    C. Are rare
    D. Are associated with pulmonary atresia
    E. Are associated with a ventricular septal defect

286. Brightly echogenic bowel may be associated with:

    A. Turner's syndrome
  — B. Down's syndrome
    C. Classic Potter's syndrome
    D. Fetal alcohol syndrome
    E. Duodenal atresia

287. Sonographic findings of a thickened nuchal fold, shortened femurs, and hypoplasia of the middle phalanx of the fifth digit are most likely associated with:

    A. Trisomy 13
    B. Trisomy 18
  — C. Trisomy 21
    D. Triploidy
    E. Turner's syndrome

288. In this image of the fetal profile, what is the arrow pointing to?

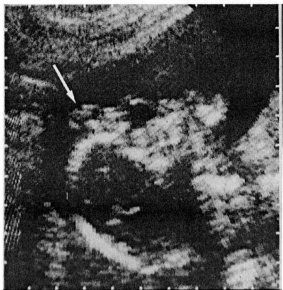

   A. Micrognathia   *small jaw*
  — B. Proboscis   *elongated nose*
   C. Macrosomia
   D. Hypospadias   *opening of urethra is on underside of penis*
   E. Macrocephaly

289. This finding would most likely be associated with:

   A. Median cleft face syndrome
   B. Lingual dermoid cyst syndrome
  — C. Beckwith-Wiedemann syndrome
   D. Fetal oral teratoma
   E. Proptosis

290. Which of the following is NOT compatible with life?

   A. Noonan's syndrome
  — B. Classic Potter's syndrome
   C. Down's syndrome
   D. Stein-Leventhal syndrome
   E. Turner's syndrome

291. Fetuses with Turner's syndrome may also have an associated:

   A. Congenital heart defect
   B. Sacrococcygeal teratoma
   C. Diaphragmatic hernia
  — D. Cystic hygroma
   E. Encephalocele

292. This image shows a common indicator for which fetal abnormality?

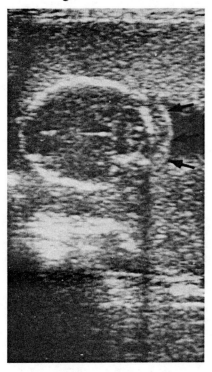

   A. Trisomy 13
   B. Trisomy 18
— C. Trisomy 21
   D. Triploidy
   E. Turner's syndrome

293. Which of these syndromes is associated with an extra set of chromosomes?

   A. Trisomy 13
   B. Trisomy 18
   C. Trisomy 21
— D. Triploidy
   E. None of the above

294. Which of these statements about Turner's syndrome is TRUE?

   A. Cystic hygroma, flat nasal profile, and webbed neck
— B. Cystic hygroma, webbed neck, and infantile sexual characteristics
   C. Flat nasal profile, duodenal atresia, and echogenic bowel
   D. Flat nasal profile, duodenal atresia, ventriculomegaly, and echogenic bowel
   E. Short stature, infantile sexual characteristics, and ventriculomegaly

295. Which of these characteristics are typical of a fetus with trisomy 21?

   A. Cystic hygroma, flat nasal profile, and webbed neck
   B. Cystic hygroma, webbed neck, and infantile sexual characteristics
   C. Flat nasal profile, duodenal atresia, and echogenic bowel
— D. Flat nasal profile, duodenal atresia, ventriculomegaly, and echogenic bowel

E. Short stature, infantile sexual characteristics, and ventriculomegaly

296. Polyhydramnios is associated with all of the following EXCEPT:

    A. Neural tube defects
  — B. Potter's syndrome
    C. Thanatophoric dwarfism
    D. GI tract obstruction
    E. Cleft lip

297. Of the following, which is NOT an indication of fetal hydrops?

    A. Anasarca
    B. Umbilical vein thrombosis
    C. Rh isoimmunization
    D. Twin to twin transfusion
  — E. Spalding's sign

298. What is *anasarca*?

    A. Scalp cyst
  — B. Skin edema
    C. Overlapping of cranial bones
    D. Overlapping of the digits
    E. Fetal decay

299. The MSAFP will be elevated with all of the following EXCEPT:

    A. Multiple gestation
    B. Anencephaly
    C. Omphalocele
  — D. Trophoblastic disease
    E. Spina bifida

300. Which of the following is NOT associated with intrauterine growth restriction (IUGR)?

    A. Placental insufficiency
    B. <10th percentile for growth
    C. Twin-to-twin transfusion
  — D. Gestational diabetic
    E. Chronic maternal hypertension

301. When intrauterine growth restriction (IUGR) is suspected due to placental insufficiency, which of the following would be useful?

    A. BHCG
    B. LS/PG
  — C. S/D ratio
    D. MSAFP
    E. None of the above

302. Given these three images, the most likely diagnosis is:

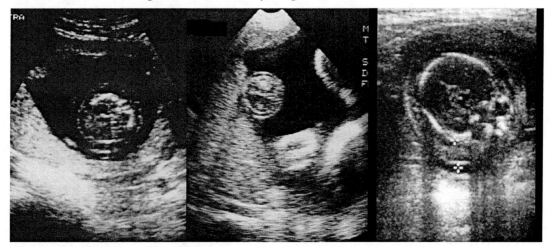

   A. Fetal demise
   B. Fetal ascites
— C. Fetal hydrops
   D. Polyhydramnios
   E. Premature rupture of membranes

COEXISTING DISORDERS [0–3%]

Leiomyoma

Cystic

Trophoblastic disease

Solid/mixed

Myometrial contraction

Other

303. A 26-year-old presents with a positive pregnancy test and right lower quadrant pain. A mass is palpated on pelvic exam. These images most likely represent:

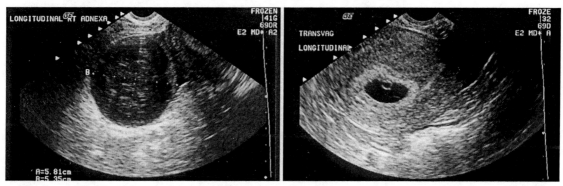

   A. Ectopic pregnancy

B. IUP with hemorrhagic cyst

C. IUP with dermoid

D. Appendicitis and IUP

E. Bicornuate uterus with IUP

304. Your patient presents at 14 weeks LMP large for gestational age and bleeding. Heart tones cannot be heard. You suspect:

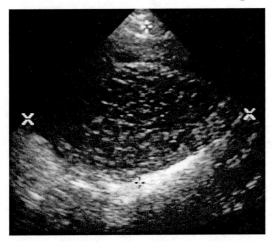

A. Fetal demise

B. Premature rupture of membranes

C. Hydatidiform mole

D. Placenta previa

E. Placental abruption

305. This patient's fundal height measured 28 cm. By good menstrual dates she should be 25 weeks. The arrow in the following longitudinal scan is pointing to:

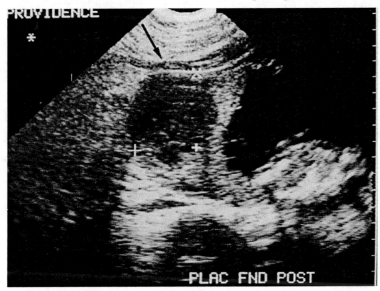

A. Uterine fibroid

B. Placental abruption

C. Chorioangioma

D. Twin abdomen

E. Ovarian cyst

306. Corpus luteal cysts accompany early pregnancy. These should resolve by:

   A. 8 weeks
   B. 10 weeks
   C. 12 weeks
   D. 14 weeks
— E. 16 weeks

307. All of the following might cause a patient to present large for gestational age EXCEPT:

   A. Uterine fibroids
   B. Polyhydramnios
— C. Fetal demise
   D. Adnexal masses
   E. Multiple gestation

308. If a pelvic mass requires surgical intervention during pregnancy, the best time to operate would be:

   A. 6–8 weeks
   B. 10–12 weeks
— C. 16–20 weeks
   D. 24–32 weeks
   E. At term

309. Of the following choices, which is considered the most common solid mass associated with pregnancy?

— A. Leiomyoma
   B. Ovarian fibroma
   C. Benign cystic teratoma
   D. Chorioangioma
   E. Endometrioma

310. Of the following choices, the most common cystic mass associated with pregnancy is:

   A. Paraovarian
— B. Corpus luteum cyst
   C. Follicular cyst
   D. Cystadenoma
   E. Theca lutein cyst

311. The adnexal finding most likely to be associated with trophoblastic disease is:

   A. Heterotopic pregnancy
   B. Polycystic ovaries

     C. Tubo-ovarian abscess

     D. Endometrioma

— E. Theca lutein cysts

312. The uterine contractions commonly seen during obstetrical sonograms are:

     A. Braxton-Hicks contractions

     B. Diffuse endometrial contractions

— C. Focal myometrial contractions

     D. Fitz-Hugh Curtis contractions

     E. Labor contractions

PART II

Gynecology

Normal Pelvic Anatomy

Physiology

Pediatric

Infertility/Endocrinology

Postmenopausal

Pelvic Pathology

Extrapelvic Pathology Associated with Gynecology

NORMAL PELVIC ANATOMY [10–15%]

Normal pelvic anatomy (uterus—corpus, endometrium, cervix, vagina)

Ovaries

Fallopian tubes

Supporting structures

Cul-de-sac

Vasculature

Doppler flow

Gynecology related studies (gastrointestinal, genitourinary)

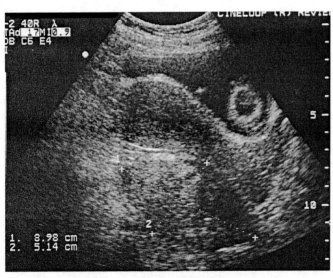

Refer to this image for questions 313–315.

313. The structure visible within the bladder in the preceding longitudinal scan most likely represents a/an:

    A. Foley catheter
    B. Ureterocele
    C. Bladder diverticulum
    D. Bladder tumor
    E. Artifact

314. Referring to the same image, how would you describe the mass being measured behind the uterus?

    A. Cystic
    B. Solid
    C. Solid but hypoechoic
    D. Complex
    E. Containing thick fluid

315. This mass is located in which pelvic space?

    A. Space of Retzius
    B. Anterior cul-de-sac
    C. Pouch of Douglas
    D. Morison's pouch
    E. Fornix

316. The menstrual cycle is influenced by all of the following EXCEPT:

    A. Hypothalamus
    B. Pituitary
    C. Ovaries
    D. Adrenal
    E. A and D

317. Which is NOT a part of the fallopian tube?

    A. Interstitial
    B. Isthmus
    C. Ampulla
    D. Infundibulum
    E. Piriformis

318. The muscles most frequently mistaken for enlarged ovaries are the:

    A. Obturator internus
    B. Piriformis
    C. Iliopsoas
    D. Levator ani
    E. Coccygeus

319. Fertilization usually occurs:

    A. In the uterus
    B. In the cornua
    C. In the isthmus
    D. In the ampulla
    E. In the fimbria

320. If a 24-year-old female shows a multilayered endometrium measuring 8 mm, she is probably:

    A. Mid cycle
    B. Menstruating
    C. Pregnant
    D. Menopausal
    E. Bleeding

321. Estrogen is responsible for all of the following EXCEPT:

    A. Stimulating endometrial proliferation
    B. Inducing rhythmic contraction of the fallopian tubes
    C. Causing fibroids to enlarge
    D. Breast duct engorgement
    E. Premenstrual syndrome

322. The floor of the pelvis is formed by the:

    A. Piriformis muscles
    B. Iliopsoas muscles
    C. Levator ani muscles
    D. Obturator internus muscles
    E. Coccygeal muscles

323. Miss Greenfield is 73 years old and asymptomatic. She is not on hormone replacement therapy. Her endometrium should not measure more than:

    A. 1 mm
    B. 2 mm
    C. 3 mm
    D. 4 mm
    E. 5 mm

324. Which vessel provides the best landmark for localizing the ovary?

    A. Common iliac artery
    B. Internal iliac artery
    C. External iliac artery
    D. Internal iliac vein
    E. External iliac vein

325. Doppler waveforms of the uterine arterial flow typically show:

    A. Low-velocity, high-resistance pattern
    B. High-velocity, low-resistance pattern
    C. High-velocity, high-resistance pattern
    D. Low-velocity, low-resistance pattern
    E. Reverse-flow pattern

326. Doppler waveforms of the ovarian arterial flow in a premenopausal woman typically show:

    A. Low-velocity, high-resistance pattern
    B. High-velocity, low-resistance pattern
    C. High-velocity, high-resistance pattern
    D. Low-velocity, low-resistance pattern
    E. Reverse-flow pattern

327. Embryologically, which system develops at the same time as the uterus?

    A. Urinary tract
    B. Gastrointestinal tract
    C. Central nervous system
    D. Skeletal system
    E. Cardiovascular system

328. Using the International Reference Preparation for hCG, which of the following levels should allow us to see an intrauterine gestational sac transabdominally?

    A. 1200
    B. 1800
    C. 2500
    D. 3000
    E. 3600

329. Using the 2nd International Standard, which of the following levels should allow us to see a normal intrauterine gestational sac transabdominally?

    A. 1200
    B. 1800
    C. 2500
    D. 3000
    E. 3600

330. Which term best describes the ovary in this image?

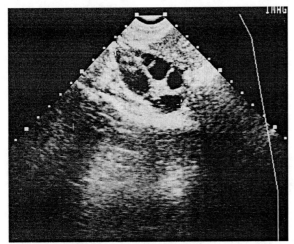

   A. Polycystic
   B. Stein-Leventhal
   C. Hyperstimulated
   D. Normal follicles
   E. Dysplastic

331. A Gartner's duct cyst is found in the:

   A. Vagina
   B. Cervix
   C. Fallopian tube
   D. Broad ligament
   E. Myometrium

332. Which of the following muscle groups form the lateral pelvic sidewalls?

   A. Iliopsoas
   B. Obturator internus
   C. Piriformis
   D. Coccygeus
   E. Levator ani

333. When the urinary bladder is empty, the uterus is normally:

   A. Anteverted
   B. Anteflexed
   C. Retroverted
   D. Retroflexed
   E. Inverted

334. The lavator ani muscles are seen, transversely, at the same level as the:

   A. Ovaries
   B. Uterine corpus

C. Cervix
D. Vagina
E. Iliac vessels

335. Which of the following is not considered a layer of the uterus?

A. Perimetrium
B. Serosa
C. Endometrium
D. Myometrium
E. Parietalis

336. Which of the following statements is TRUE of nabothian cysts?

A. They are a common cause for infertility.
A. They predispose patients to develop cervical cancer.
B. They are benign, common, and frequently multiple.
C. They are uncommon in postmenopausal patients.
D. They are clinically significant and require immediate intervention.

337. The iliac vessels usually lie _____ to the ovaries.

A. Anterior
B. Superior
C. Lateral
D. Medial
E. Inferior

338. Which of the following statements is NOT true of the fallopian tubes?

A. They lie within the broad ligament.
B. Fertilization usually occurs within the ampullary portion.
C. The tube provides nutrients for the ova.
D. Fallopian tubes are routinely imaged sonographically.
E. The fimbria communicates with the peritoneal cavity.

339. This was discovered during transvaginal evaluation of the pelvis. The patient was asymptomatic. You suspect:

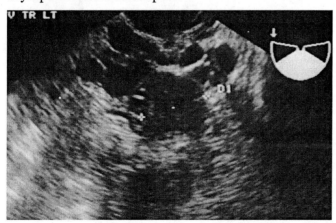

A. Dilated fallopian tube
B. Hydrosalpinx
C. Dilated veins
D. Dilated ureter
E. Septated mass

340. Sonographically, how will the uterus of a nulliparous female appear compared to that of a multiparous female?

A. Smaller
B. Larger
C. More dense
D. Flatter
E. More globular

341. The ovaries of a patient who has had a bilateral salpingo-oophorectomy will appear:

A. Enlarged
B. Atrophied
C. Nonvisualized
D. Prominent but normal
E. Normal

342. Anatomically, the uterus lies _____ to the urinary bladder and _____ to the rectum:

A. Lateral, medial
B. Medial, lateral
C. Anterior, posterior
D. Posterior, anterior
E. Superior, inferior

343. Choose the statement that most accurately describes the anatomic relationships among the ureter, ovary, and iliac vessels:

A. The ureter is posterior to the ovary, and the iliac vessels are anterior.
B. The ureter is anterior to the ovary, and the iliac vessels are posterior.
C. The ureter and iliac vessels are anterior to the ovary.
D. The ureter and iliac vessels are posterior to the ovary.
E. The ureter and iliac vessels are medial to the ovary.

344. The true pelvis includes all of the following structures except:

A. Bladder
B. Uterus
C. Ovaries
D. Fallopian tubes
E. Bowel

345. Your patient is 21 years old and is a nulligravida. Her uterus, if normal, should measure:

   A. 9 x 7 x 6 cm
   B. 8 x 3 x 4 cm
   C. 4 x 3 x 3 cm
   D. 10 x 4 x 6 cm
   E. 11 x 2 x 3 cm

346. Embryologically, the _____ ducts fuse to form the uterus, vagina, and fallopian tubes.

   A. Mesonephric
   B. Wolffian
   C. Gonadal
   D. Primordial
   E. Mullerian

347. Which of these patients would not be a good candidate for a transvaginal exam?

   A. Patient with a possible ectopic pregnancy
   B. Patient with a threatened abortion
   C. Patient with an adnexal mass
   D. Patient with a large fibroid uterus
   E. Patient who is morbidly obese and postmenopausal

348. All of the following statements about transvaginal sonography are true EXCEPT:

   A. Resolution is improved by use of higher frequencies.
   B. Does not require a full bladder technique.
   C. Can penetrate up to 12 cm depth.
   D. Can identify an intrauterine pregnancy at 4–5 weeks.
   E. Is contraindicated in virginal patients.

349. Which of these agents is NOT considered satisfactory for use as a disinfectant for the vaginal transducer?

   A. Betadine
   B. Bleach
   C. Cidex
   D. Sporicidin
   E. Transeptic

   The image on the following page applies to questions 350 and 351.

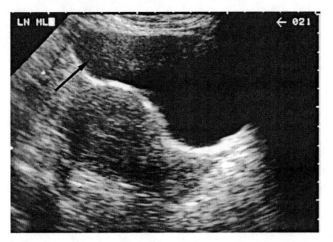

350. Which term best describes the appearance of this uterus?

    A. Normal
    B. Globular
    C. Anteflexed
    D. Atrophied
    E. Infantile

351. To what, in the bladder, is the arrow pointing?

    A. Thickened bladder wall
    B. Debris within the bladder
    C. Anterior reverberation artifact
    D. Cystitis
    E. Bladder flap hematoma

352. To what is the arrow pointing in this transverse image?

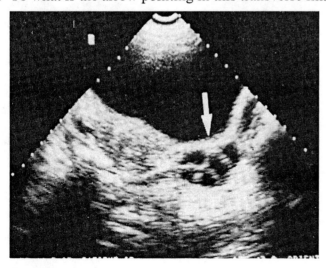

    A. Uterus
    B. Right ovary
    C. Left ovary
    D. Broad ligament
    E. Muscle

353. Which term best describes the appearance of the ovary in the previous image?

    A. Normal
    B. Hyperstimulated
    C. Polycystic
    D. Hydropic
    E. Obstructed

354. In this sagittal transvaginal image of the ovary the arrow is pointing to:

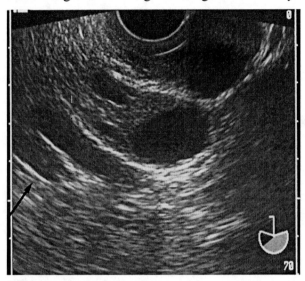

    A. Internal iliac artery
    B. Internal iliac vein
    C. Dilated ureter
    D. Hydrosalpinx
    E. Fluid-filled bowel

355. Describe the position of the uterus from this sagittal transvaginal image.

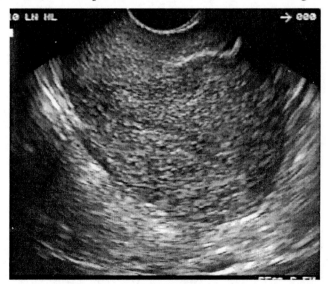

A. Dextroposed
B. Levoposed
C. Anteflexed
D. Retroflexed
E. Prolapsed

356. Which part of the uterus is the least distinctive part?

A. Isthmus
B. Corpus
C. Fundus
D. Cervix
E. Body

357. All of these statements about the broad ligament are true EXCEPT:

A. It is not a true ligament.
B. It divides the true pelvis into anterior and posterior compartments.
C. The ovaries attach to the posterior surface.
D. It is a major suspensory ligament for the uterus.
E. It can be seen when there is pelvic ascites.

358. *Hypogastric artery* is another name for the:

A. Right common iliac artery
B. Left common iliac artery
C. External iliac artery
D. Internal iliac artery
E. Femoral artery

359. For Doppler evaluation of the uterine artery, insonation at the following level provides the best access to the vessel:

A. Cervical
B. Isthmus
C. Cornual
D. Body
E. Fundal

360. The potential space around the cervix is called the:

A. Pouch of Douglas
B. Morrison's pouch
C. Anterior cul-de-sac
D. Space of Retzius
E. Fornix

361. What maneuver would best improve the quality of this longitudinal image through the uterus?

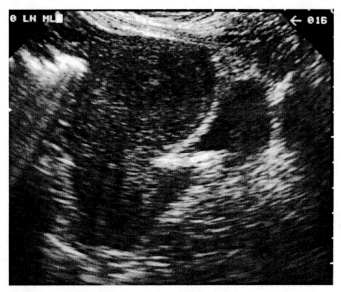

A. Fill the bladder.
B. Increase overall gain.
C. Decrease overall gain.
D. Adjust TGC.
E. Do a transvaginal exam.

The following image applies to questions 362–364.

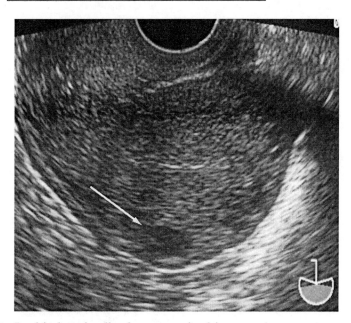

362. In this longitudinal transvaginal image, the appearance of the endometrium is best characterized as:

A. Proliferative
B. Preovulatory
C. Periovulatory
D. Secretory
E. Decidualized

363. The arrow in this image is pointing to what most likely is a/an:

    A. Arcuate vessel
    B. Myometrial cyst
    C. Leiomyoma
    D. Artifact
    E. Endometrioma

364. The structure mentioned above is located in the:

    A. Posterior myometrium
    B. Anterior myometrium
    C. Fundus of the uterus
    D. Cervix of the uterus
    E. Isthmus of the uterus

The following image applies to questions 365 and 366.

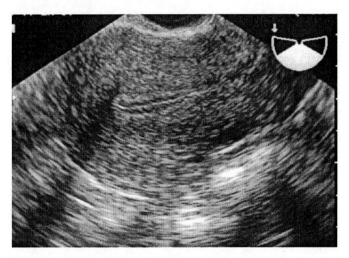

365. Which phase of the menstrual cycle is this patient in?

    A. Proliferative
    B. Secretory
    C. Periovulatory
    D. Late menstrual
    E. Perimenopausal

366. The position of the uterus in this transvaginal image is:

    A. Dextroposed
    B. Levoposed
    C. Retroflexed
    D. Anteflexed
    E. Retroverted

367. The arrows in this transverse image point to:

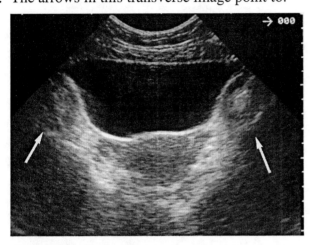

    A. Enlarged ovaries
    B. Benign cystic teratomas
    C. Kruckenburg's tumors
    D. Pelvic bones
    E. Iliopsoas muscles

368. Which part of the uterus is indicated by the arrow?

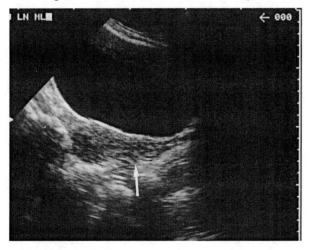

    A. Corpus
    B. Fundus
    C. Isthmus
    D. Cervix
    E. Vagina

369. A mature follicle ready for ovulation is referred to as the:

    A. Corpus luteum
    B. Graafian follicle
    C. Corpus albicans
    D. Preantral follicle
    E. Theca lutein

PHYSIOLOGY [6–15%]

Menstrual cycle

Pregnancy tests

Human chorionic gonadotropin (hCG)

Fertilization

370. Ovulation usually occurs when the dominant follicle reaches the following size:

    A. 10 mm
    B. 15 mm
    C. 1.5 cm
    D. 2.5 cm
    E. 3.5 cm

371. A 24-year-old patient at day 14 of her menstrual cycle should show a _____ endometrium:

    A. Proliferative
    B. Periovulatory
    C. Secretory
    D. Decidualized
    E. Menstrual

372. Fertilization usually occurs _____ hours after ovulation:

    A. 4–8
    B. 8–12
    C. 12–24
    D. 24–36
    E. 36–48

373. All of the following are considered physiologic conditions of the ovary EXCEPT:

    A. Follicular cyst
    B. Corpus luteal cyst
    C. Dermoid cyst
    D. Theca lutein cyst
    E. Polycystic ovaries

374. Endometrial proliferation is stimulated by:

    A. Human choriogonadotropin
    B. Progesterone
    C. Testosterone
    D. Alpha-fetoprotein
    E. Estrogen

375. If the 2nd International Standard for hCG is 2000, the IRP level would be:

    A. 1000
    B. 2000
    C. 3000
    D. 4000
    E. 5000

376. The _____ level rises to produce a positive pregnancy test:

    A. Human choriogonadotropin (hCG)
    B. Alpha-fetoprotein (AFP)
    C. Follicle stimulating hormone (FSH)
    D. Luteinizing hormone (LH)
    E. Amniotic fluid index (AFI)

377. A patient is taking oral contraceptives would not be expected to develop a:

    A. Follicular cyst
    B. Corpus luteal cyst
    C. Nabothian cyst
    D. Paraovarian cyst
    E. Gartner's duct cyst

378. The term used to describe the onset of the first menstrual cycle is:

    A. Dysmenorrhea
    B. Amenorrhea
    C. Menopausal
    D. Menarche
    E. Menses

379. The endometrial echo would appear hypoechoic:

    A. During the secretory phase of the menstrual cycle
    B. After dilatation and curettage
    C. After insertion of an intrauterine device
    D. During the periovulatory stage
    E. Upon decidualization

380. Until ovulation, ovarian follicles grow at the daily rate of:

    A. 1–2 mm

B. 2–3 mm
C. 3–4 mm
D. 4–5 mm
E. 5–6 mm

381. The phase of the menstrual cycle following ovulation is referred to as the:

    A. Proliferative phase
    B. Periovulatory phase
    C. Preovulatory phase
    D. Menstrual phase
    E. Secretory phase

382. How soon after conception will pregnancy tests produce positive results?

    A. 1–2 weeks
    B. 2–3 weeks
    C. 3–4 weeks
    D. 4–5 weeks
    E. 5–6 weeks

383. This method of birth control is virtually 100% effective in preventing pregnancy:

    A. Spermicidal foam
    B. Rhythm method
    C. Combination oral contraceptives
    D. Intrauterine contraceptive devices
    E. Condoms

384. A fertilized egg is called the:

    A. Morula
    B. Zygote
    C. Blastocyst
    D. Gestational sac
    E. Primary yolk sac

385. Follicle stimulating hormone (FSH) is produced by the:

    A. Ovary
    B. Corpus luteum
    C. Hypothalamus
    D. Pituitary
    E. Thyroid

386. When monitoring the hormone levels during early pregnancy, normal hCG levels should double every:

    A. 12 hours
    B. 24 hours
    C. 48 hours

D. 36 hours

E. 72 hours

387. The 2nd International Standard for hCG is _____ the International Reference Preparation level (IRP).

A. One-fourth

B. One-third

C. One-half

D. Double

E. Triple

388. The hCG titers associated with an ectopic pregnancy:

A. Increase to a point and then plateau

B. Are lower than normal

C. Increase to extremely high levels

D. Are inadequate in determining pregnancy

E. Are no different from those of a normal pregnancy

389. If a 30-year-old female is on day 8 of her menstrual cycle and she has normal regular periods, her endometrium should measure:

A. 4 mm

B. 6 mm

C. 8 mm

D. 10 mm

E. 12 mm

390. If you discover an ovarian cyst measuring 2.5 cm in a 23-year-old female, what finding would suggest to you that this cyst is a dominant follicle rather than a corpus luteum cyst?

A. Cul-de-sac fluid

B. Debris within the cyst

C. Clean smooth walls

D. Fibrinous strands within

E. Thick walls

391. The normal menstrual cycle occurs every:

A. 20 days

B. 24 days

C. 28 days

D. 32 days

E. 40 days

392. The hormone responsible for inducing ovulation during the normal menstrual cycle is:

A. LH

B. FSH
C. Estrogen
D. Progesterone
E. PAPPA

393. The hormone mostly responsible for premenstrual symptoms and those of early pregnancy is:

A. LH
B. FSH
C. Estrogen
D. Progesterone
E. PAPPA

394. The phase of the menstrual cycle when the endometrium is its thinnest is the:

A. Secretory phase
B. Periovulatory phase
C. Preovulatory phase
D. Luteal phase
E. Proliferative phase

395. The term that refers to mid-cycle or ovulatory pain is:

A. Dysmenorrhea
B. Dyspareunia
C. Mittleschmertz
D. Menstrual distress
E. Premenstrual syndrome

396. Human choriogonadotropin (hCG) is produced by the:

A. Fetal liver
B. Fetal kidneys
C. Maternal ovaries
D. Placenta
E. Yolk sac

397. If a patient relates a history of normal menses every 28 days, on which day of her cycle should ovulation occur?

A. 7
B. 14
C. 21
D. 28
E. 30

398. Which of the following is NOT considered a physiologic condition of the ovary?

A. Corpus luteum cyst
B. Theca lutein cyst

C. Follicular cyst

D. Polycystic ovaries

E. Cystadenoma

399. In the female, circulating testosterone is derived mostly from:

A. Liver, ovary, and skin

B. Liver and skin

C. Ovary and adrenal gland

D. Adrenal gland

E. All of the above

400. The term for absence of menses is:

A. Amenorrhea

B. Dysmenorrhea

C. Menorrhagia

D. Agenesis

E. Metrorrhagia

401. The normal cessation of menses is called:

A. Menopause

B. Menarche

C. Menstruation

D. Mensation

E. Mittlepause

402. Based on this sagittal transvaginal image of the uterus, you suspect the patient to be in this phase of the menstrual cycle:

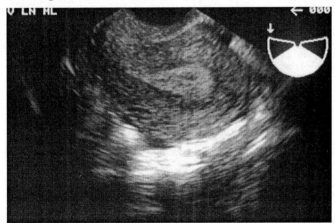

A. Proliferative

B. Preovulatory

C. Periovulatory

D. Secretory

E. Mid cycle

403. In the same image, the position of the uterus is best described as:

    A. Anteflexed
    B. Retroflexed
    C. Dextroposed
    D. Levoposed
    E. Prolapsed

404. This image of the adnexa of a patient at day 20 in her menstrual cycle is consistent with a:

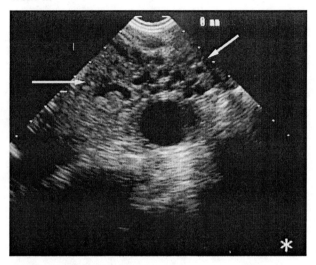

    A. Follicular cyst
    B. Corpus luteum cyst
    C. Dermoid cyst
    D. Theca lutein cyst
    E. Neoplastic cyst

405. In the same image, the arrows points to:

    A. Hydrosalpinx
    B. Endometriosis
    C. Pyosalpinx
    D. Engorged vessels
    E. Fluid filled bowel

406. The influence of the follicle stimulating hormone (FSH) and luteinizing hormone (LH) are required for normal oogenesis. These hormones are produced by the:

    A. Ovaries
    B. Adrenal glands
    C. Hypothalamus
    D. Thymus
    E. Pituitary gland

407. In the absence of fertilization, the corpus luteum cyst should regress after:

    A. 4 days
    B. 8 days
    C. 10 days
    D. 14 days

PEDIATRIC [1–5%]

    Precocious puberty

    Hematometra/hematocolpos

    Sexual ambiguity

    Other

408. A 12-year-old patient presents with primary amenorrhea and pelvic pressure. The most likely cause for her symptoms is:

    A. Pregnancy
    B. Leiomyoma
    C. Cystic teratoma
    D. Pelvic inflammatory disease
    E. Hematocolpos

409. Female pseudohermaphroditism is most often caused by:

    A. Failure of the mullerian ducts to fuse
    B. Testicular feminization
    C. Ovarian masculinization
    D. Adrenal hyperplasia
    E. Pituitary imbalance

410. A 13-year-old female presents with lower abdominal pain and pressure. On the basis of this longitudinal image through the uterus you suspect:

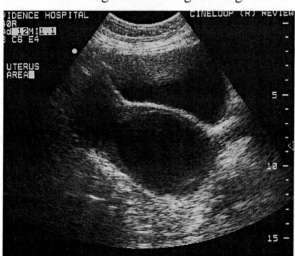

A. Hematocolpos
B. Hematometracolpos
C. Hematosalpinx
D. Hematoma
E. Hematoperitoneum

411. The most likely cause for this condition is:

   A. Cervical cancer
   B. Endometrial cancer
   C. Imperforate hymen
   D. Vaginal agenesis
   E. Turner's syndrome

412. Which of the following conditions is the most common among pediatric patients?

   A. Pelvic inflammatory disease
   B. Endometriosis
   C. Cervical carcinoma
   D. Sarcoma botroyoid
   E. Cystadenoma

413. Which of the following ovarian tumors would cause precocious puberty in a child?

   A. Benign cystic teratoma
   B. Cystadenoma
   C. Arrhenoblastoma
   D. Granulosa cell tumor
   E. Sertoli-Leydig tumor

414. The most common cause for gonadal dysgenesis is:

   A. Sertoli-Leydig tumor
   B. Stein-Leventhal syndrome
   C. Polycystic ovary disease
   D. Precocious puberty
   E. Turner's syndrome

415. Which statement is TRUE for an infantile uterus?

   A. The size and shape remains constant throughout life.
   B. The corpus and fundus are the most prominent portions of the uterus.
   C. The cervix occupies most of the length of the uterine body until puberty.
   D. Pubertal changes cause the uterus to atrophy and the ovaries to enlarge.
   E. Transvaginal sonography is the best technique for visualization.

416. Which of the following conditions is associated with sexual ambiguity?

    A. Mixed gonadal dysgenesis
    B. Pure gonadal dysgenesis
    C. Testicular feminization
    D. Turner's syndrome
    E. Noonan's syndrome

INFERTILITY / ENDOCRINOLOGY [2–6%]

Contraception

Causes

Medications and treatment

Ovulation induction (follicular monitoring)

ART (assisted reproductive technology)—GIFT, IVF, ZIFT

/ /

417. This image demonstrates that the cause of the patient's infertility is:

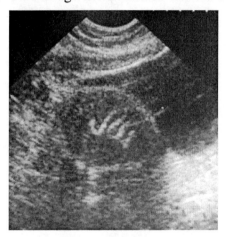

    A. Calcified endometrium
    B. Endometrial agenesis
    C. Intrauterine device
    D. Normal endometrial echo appearance
    E. Endometrial cysts

418. The most common cause(s) of infertility among couples is/are:

    A. Tubal damage
    B. Endometriosis
    C. Sperm failure
    D. Ovulatory failure
    E. All of the above

419. The failure to ovulate is termed:

    A. Oocyte
    B. Anovulation
    C. Amenorrhea
    D. Ovulatory agenesis
    E. Ovarian cycle

420. The most common procedure for determining if fallopian tubes have been compromised during some event, causing infertility?

    A. Endoscopic surgery
    B. Sonohysterography
    C. Fluoroscopy
    D. Hysterosalpingography
    E. Endoscopy

421. This image of a patient who presents with right lower quadrant pain demonstrates:

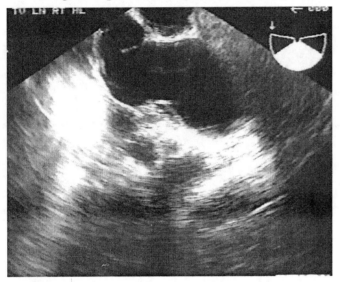

    A. Fecaloma
    B. Appendix
    C. Pelvic kidney
    D. Hydrosalpinx
    E. Bowel gas

422. It is estimated that 40% of women with the following problem will have trouble conceiving:

    A. Adenomyosis
    B. Salpingitis
    C. Endometriosis
    D. Endometritis
    E. Leiomyomatosis

423. *Postcoital* means:

    A. After stimulation
    B. After pregnancy
    C. After childbirth
    D. After sexual intercourse
    E. After induction

424. What hormone in the female body stimulates cervical mucus production?

    A. Progesterone
    B. Testosterone
    C. Estrogen
    D. Estradiol
    E. Luteinizing hormone
    F. Follicular stimulating hormone

425. The sonographic appearance of the endometrium in this image indicates which phase of the menstrual cycle?

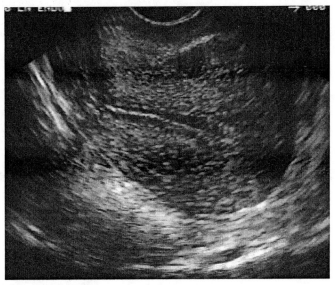

    A. Preovulatory
    B. Early gestation
    C. Postovulatory
    D. Secretory
    E. Proliferative

426. Sonohysterography is a common procedure used to determine some causes of infertility, including:

    A. Endometriosis
    B. Endometrial polyp
    C. Adenomyosis
    D. A and B
    E. All of the above

427. The drug of choice most commonly used to induce ovulation is:

    A. hCG
    B. Pergonal
    C. Falastem
    D. FSH
    E. Clomid

428. A hormone used to trigger ovulation is:

    A. hCG
    B. Pergonal
    C. Falastem
    D. FSH
    E. Clomid

429. The advantages of transvaginal over transabdominal ultrasound when tracking follicular development include all of the following EXCEPT:

    A. More precise information
    B. Better resolution
    C. Greater comfort
    D. No preparation
    E. Limited field of view

430. The most common complication related to pharmaceutical stimulation of follicular growth is:

    A. Death
    B. Failure
    C. Anovulation
    D. Hyperstimulation
    E. Dysmenorrhea

431. What lab value is compared to the ultrasound findings to determine when the ovary is ready to ovulate?

    A. Estrotest
    B. Estradiol
    C. hCG
    D. FSH
    E. LH

432. In vitro fertilization:

    A. Permits the physician to retrieve many oocytes
    B. Is performed when the tube is not obstructed
    C. Allows the physician to retrieve only one oocyte
    D. Decreases the number of embryos to be implanted
    E. Does not require ultrasound guidance

433. Which of the following is true about GIFT?

    A. GIFT is gamete intrafallopian transfer.
    B. Both tubes must be normal.
    C. GIFT has a higher incidence of success than in vitro fertilization (IVF).
    D. A and B
    E. A and C

434. A procedure involving the transfer of fertilized oocytes into the fallopian tube either laparoscopically or transcervically is:

    A. GIFT
    B. IVF
    C. ZIFT
    D. DES
    E. OHS

POSTMENOPAUSAL [6–10%]

    Anatomy

    Physiology

    Therapy (hormonal replacement)

    Pathology (hyperplasia, polyps, endometrial cancer, ovarian cancer, other)

435. Which of the following statements is true for postmenopausal patients?

    A. Endometrial fluid collections are common.
    B. Postmenopausal ovaries frequently exhibit follicles.
    C. Uterine size and echogenicity increase with age.
    D. Endometrial cancer is the most common cause of postmenopausal bleeding.
    E. Hormone replacement therapy decreases one's chances of developing endometrial cancer.

436. The normal endometrium of a postmenopausal patient is usually:

    A. Hypoechoic
    B. Multi-layered
    C. Thick and hyperechoic
    D. Thin
    E. Cystic

437. The endometrium of a patient receiving hormone replacement therapy would be considered abnormal if it measured more than:

    A. 1 mm
    B. 3 mm

    C. 5 mm
    D. 6 mm
    E. 8 mm

438. Miss Crenshaw is 74 years old and is not taking hormones. Her endometrium should not measure more than:

    A. 1 mm
    B. 3 mm
    C. 5 mm
    D. 6 mm
    E. 8 mm

439. Which statement is NOT true of postmenopausal ovaries?

    A. They should measure less than 2 cm in their greatest dimension.
    B. They should not exceed 8 cubic centimeters in volume each.
    C. They can be recognized by the multiple echogenic foci within them.
    D. They can always be identified transvaginally.
    E. The incidence of ovarian cancer is higher in postmenopausal patients.

440. An 85-year-old female is having postmenopausal bleeding. This longitudinal image suggests:

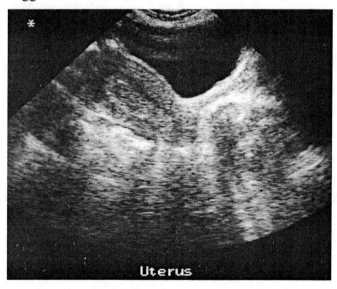

    A. Fibroids
    B. Adenomyosis
    C. Endometrial carcinoma
    D. Endometrial polyps
    E. Endometritis

441. The most common cause for postmenopausal bleeding is:

    A. Benign hyperplasia
    B. Endometrial polyps

C. Endometritis

D. Endometrial carcinoma

E. Cervical cancer

442. Which of the following disease processes should NOT be seen in the postmenopausal patient?

A. Endometrial carcinoma

B. Ovarian cancer

C. Endometrial hyperplasia

— D. Endometriosis

E. Leiomyomas

443. Which of the following is considered the most common gynecologic malignancy in the United States?

A. Cervical

— B. Endometrial

C. Ovarian

D. Tubal

E. Bladder

444. Of the following statements, which is TRUEST for the postmenopausal uterus?

— A. It decreases in size and is infantile in appearance.

B. It becomes hypoechoic and globular.

C. The endometrium becomes calcific.

D. The ovaries become more prominent than the uterine corpus.

E. It undergoes autohysterectomy.

445. On color Doppler sonography, most malignant ovarian tumors yield flow signals that are best characterized as:

A. Avascular

B. High impedance

— C. Low impedance

D. Variable

E. No flow

446. If a postmenopausal patient is asymptomatic and fluid is identified within her endometrial cavity, the most likely cause of the fluid would be:

A. Endometrial carcinoma

B. Endometritis

C. Pelvic inflammatory disease

— D. Endometrial atrophy

E. Vesicovaginal fistula

PELVIC PATHOLOGY [6–10%]

Congenital uterine malformation

Uterine masses

Ovarian masses

Endometriosis

Polycystic ovarian disease

Inflammatory disease

Doppler flow studies

Gynecology related studies (gastrointestinal, genitourinary)

Other

//

447. An ovarian tumor accompanied by pelvic ascites usually suggests malignancy. An exception to this rule would be ascites associated with:

   A. Dysgerminoma
   B. Ovarian fibroma
   C. Pseudomyxoma peritonei
   D. Yolk sac tumor
   E. Cystadenocarcinoma

448. The most common site for an extrauterine adnexal mass is the:

   A. Ovary
   B. Fallopian tubes
   C. Cervix
   D. Broad ligament
   E. Fornix

449. All of the following are solid tumors except:

   A. Thecoma
   B. Fibroma
   C. Brenner's tumor
   D. Cystadenoma
   E. Teratoma

450. Which of these masses is considered malignant?

   A. Endometrioma
   B. Cystadenoma
   C. Dermoid
   D. Dysgerminoma
   E. Pyosalpinx

451. Most adnexal masses are:

    A. Cystic, ovarian in origin, and malignant
    B. Cystic and ovarian in origin
    C. Ovarian in origin and malignant
    D. Cystic and malignant
    E. None of the above

452. "Chocolate cyst" is a lay term for a(n):

    A. Degenerating fibroid
    B. Endometrioma
    C. Hemorrhagic cyst
    D. Tubo-ovarian abscess
    E. Ectopic pregnancy

453. In the evaluation of an adnexal mass, the following findings increase the likelihood of malignancy:

    A. Premenopausal patient with mass that measures less than 6 cm
    B. Postmenopausal patient with thin-walled, unilocular fluid-filled mass
    C. Large thick-walled cyst with multiple thick septations and free fluid
    D. Teenager with complex solid mass showing calcifications
    E. Symptomatic dilated pelvic vasculature

454. A benign cystic teratoma contains tissues from:

    A. Ectoderm
    B. Ectoderm and mesoderm
    C. Ectoderm and endoderm
    D. Ectoderm, mesoderm, and endoderm
    E. None of the above

455. A dermoid cyst contains tissues from:

    A. Ectoderm
    B. Ectoderm and mesoderm
    C. Ectoderm and endoderm
    D. Ectoderm, mesoderm, and endoderm
    E. None of the above

456. Stein-Leventhal syndrome is characterized by:

    A. Menorrhagia, obesity, and hirsutism
    B. Menorrhagia, obesity, and infertility
    C. Obesity, hirsutism, and infertility
    D. Menorrhagia, hirsutism, and infertility
    E. Menorrhagia, obesity, hirsutism, and infertility

457. A granulosa cell tumor is:

    A. Androgenic
    B. Benign
    C. Estrogenic
    D. Androgenic and benign
    E. Benign and estrogenic

458. A 52-year-old female presents as postmenopausal for 5 years, G-4-P4. Her uterus is enlarged upon palpation and is irregular in contour. You suspect:

    A. Endometrial cancer
    B. Adenomyosis
    C. Endometriosis
    D. Hydatidiform mole
    E. Leiomyoma

459. Which of these masses is considered androgenic?

    A. Fibroma
    B. Arrhenoblastoma
    C. Brenner's tumor
    D. Granulosa cell tumor
    E. Cystadenoma

460. Your patient has a suspicious adnexal neoplasm. To assist in ruling out metastasis, you scan the:

    A. Lymph nodes
    B. Liver
    C. Kidneys
    D. Spleen
    E. Breasts

461. Bicornuate uterus is a congenital malformation that results from incomplete fusion of the:

    A. Mullerian ducts
    B. Wolffian ducts
    C. Graafian ducts
    D. Bartholin ducts
    E. Gartner's ducts

462. On a transverse image of the pelvis, a complex mass is seen displacing the anterior bladder wall posteriorly. This mass is located in the:

    A. Pouch of Douglas
    B. Uterovesical space
    C. Morrison's pouch
    D. Space of Retzius
    E. Anterior cul-de-sac

463. Transvaginal evaluation reveals a large cyst in the adnexa that is separate from the ovary. It is unilocular and thin-walled. This most likely represents:

    A. Paraovarian cyst
    B. Theca lutein cyst
    C. Corpus luteum cyst
    D. Mesenteric cyst
    E. Cystadenoma

464. Which of these statements is NOT true of endometriosis?

    A. It is a disease of upper middle-class professional women.
    B. It is more common among Caucasians.
    C. There is a hereditary predisposition.
    D. Symptoms are cyclic.
    E. It is associated with multiparity.

465. Which of the following are considered symptoms for endometriosis?

    A. Menorrhagia and dysmenorrhea
    B. Dysmenorrhea and dyspareunia
    C. Menorrhagia, dysmenorrhea, and dyspareunia
    D. Menorrhagia and cyclic pain
    E. Menorrhagia, dysmenorrhea, dyspareunia, and cyclic pain

466. The most common location for a benign cystic teratoma is:

    A. Anterior and superior
    B. Posterior and inferior
    C. In the right adnexa
    D. In the left adnexa
    E. In the false pelvis

467. Which statement best describes the Kruckenburg's tumor?

    A. It is a solid, benign tumor of the ovary.
    B. It is a metastatic tumor from a GI tract primary.
    C. It is a cystic malignant tumor of the uterus
    D. A and B
    E. B and C

468. All of these statements about endometrioma are true EXCEPT:

    A. It is a malignant tumor of the endometrium.
    B. It is sometimes referred to as a "chocolate cyst."
    C. It is associated with endometriosis.
    D. It will be adnexal in location.
    E. It is usually asymptomatic.

469. Of the following, the most common benign tumor of the uterus is:

    A. Leiomyosarcoma
    B. Endometrioma
    C. Leiomyoma
    D. Adenomyosa
    E. Kruckenburg's

470. Uterine fibroids are associated with:

    A. Infertility
    B. Menstrual irregularities
    C. Back pain
    D. Frequency
    E. All of the above

471. One would not expect to see cul-de-sac fluid with:

    A. Pelvic inflammatory disease
    B. Uterine fibroids
    C. Normal ovulation
    D. Ectopic pregnancy
    E. Pelvic ascites

472. A 43-year-old female complains of lower back pain and menorrhagia. Her history and this longitudinal image suggest:

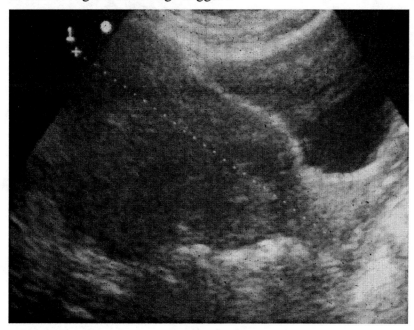

    A. Fibroid uterus
    B. Ovarian tumor
    C. Trophoblastic disease
    D. Adenomyosis

E. Endometrial carcinoma

473. A Gartner's duct cyst is found in the:

    A. Ovary
    B. Uterus
    C. Vagina
    D. Cervix
    E. Broad ligament

474. What does this transverse image demonstrate?

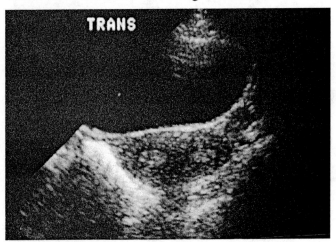

    A. Normal proliferative uterus
    B. Calcified fibroid
    C. Endometrial polyps
    D. Internal endometriosis
    E. Bicornuate uterus

    The image on the following page
    applies to questions 475 and 476.

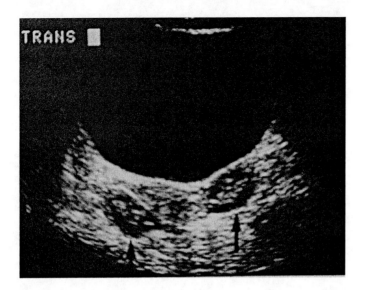

475. This patient presents with oligomenorrhea, hirsutism, and infertility. The arrows are pointing to:

    A. Uterus
    B. Ovaries
    C. Piriform muscles
    D. Fallopian tubes
    E. Bowel

476. This sonogram is typical of:

    A. Bicornuate uterus
    B. Polycystic ovaries
    C. Hypertrophied musculature
    D. Pelvic inflammatory disease
    E. Constipation

477. Your patient tests positive for chlamydia and presents with severe pelvic pain. This finding is most typical of:

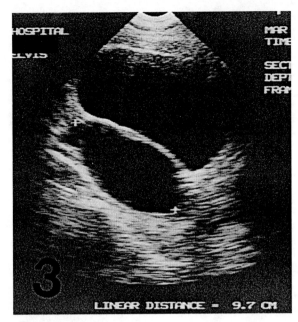

A. Hydrosalpinx
B. Hematometra
C. Ectopic pregnancy
D. Ovarian cyst
E. Appendicitis

478. All of the following could cause pelvic inflammatory disease EXCEPT:

    A. Sexually transmitted disease
    B. Ruptured appendix
    TORCH (toxoplasma, rubella, cytomegalovirus, herpes simplex virus)
    C. Exposure to DES (diethylstilbestrol)
    D. Tuberculosis

479. All of the following symptoms are consistent with uterine fibroids EXCEPT:

    A. Nausea and vomiting
    B. Menorrhagia
    C. Back pain
    D. Urinary frequency
    E. Constipation

480. Diethylstilbestrol (DES) is known to increase a patient's risk for all of the following EXCEPT:

    A. Uterine malformations
    B. Cervical cancer
    C. Multiple gestations
    D. Preterm labor
    E. Ectopic pregnancy

481. DES was prescribed to pregnant women during the 1940s and 1950s to:

    A. Inhibit spontaneous abortion
    B. Relieve morning sickness
    C. Treat trophoblastic disease
    D. Offset RH isoimmunization
    E. Relieve pain

482. Nabothian cysts are found in the:

    A. Ovary
    B. Broad ligament
    C. Cervix
    D. Vagina
    E. Fallopian tube

483. Which statement about ovarian tumors is TRUE?

    A. Most are solid.
    B. Most are malignant.
    C. Most are benign.
    D. Most develop postmenopausally.
    E. Most are seen in adolescents.

484. Which of these adnexal pathologies is associated with Meigs' syndrome?

    A. Benign cystic teratoma
    B. Ovarian fibroma
    C. Endometrioma
    D. Tubo-ovarian abscess
    E. Polycystic ovaries

485. Fitz-Hugh Curtis syndrome is associated with:

    A. Pelvic inflammatory disease
    B. Endometriosis
    C. Ovarian fibroma
    D. Polycystic ovaries
    E. Ovarian cancer

486. Fitz-Hugh Curtis syndrome consists of:

    A. Hirsutism and infertility
    B. Pelvic ascites and pleural effusion
    C. Webbed neck and gonadal dysgenesis
    D. Right upper quadrant pain and PID
    E. Pelvic ascites and metastases to the liver

487. Large pelvic masses, whether benign or malignant, may cause _____; therefore the _____ should be evaluated also:

A. Metastatic lesions, liver
B. Gallstones, gallbladder
C. Biliary obstruction, liver and biliary tree
D. Portal-splenic hypertension, liver and spleen
E. Urinary obstruction, kidneys

488. If a primary malignant process is suspected in the pelvis, one should also scan the:

A. Liver and lymph nodes
B. Lymph nodes and kidneys
C. Kidneys and pancreas
D. None of the above
E. All of the above

EXTRAPELVIC PATHOLOGY ASSOCIATED WITH GYNECOLOGY [1–3%]

Ascites

Liver metastasis

Hydronephrosis

Other

489. This patient presents in her mid second trimester with right flank pain. Her obstetrical sonogram is normal so the doctor orders an ultrasound exam of her right upper quadrant. The longitudinal scan on the following page demonstrates:

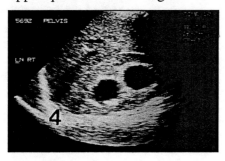

A. Gallstones
B. Cholecystitis
C. Hydronephrosis
D. Pyelonephritis
E. Liver enlargement

490. Whenever you suspect pelvic ascites, you should:

A. Have the patient void and then rescan.
B. Always check Morison's pouch.
C. Scan the liver.
D. A and B
E. B and C

491. A patient presents with abdominal swelling, low back pain, and an extremely elevated CA-125. These clinical findings suggest:

 A. Pregnancy
 B. Infection
 C. Hemorrhage
 D. Malignancy
 E. Findings are nonspecific

492. This longitudinal sonogram through the right lower quadrant of the same patient suggests:

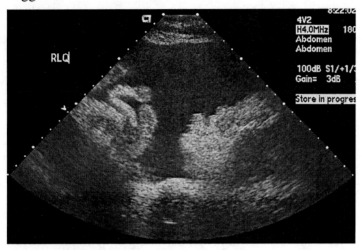

 A. Ruptured ectopic
 B. Pelvic inflammatory disease
 C. Ruptured appendix
 D. Endometriosis
 E. Pelvic ascites

493. In the same patient, evaluation of her right upper quadrant indicates:

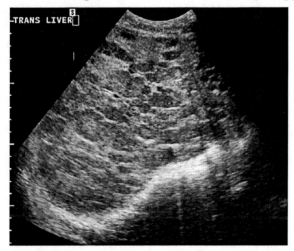

 A. Normal liver
 B. Abdominal ascites

C. Perihepatitis
D. Metastatic liver disease
E. Liver abscess

494. Perihepatitis can be associated with pelvic inflammatory disease, causing right upper quadrant tenderness and pain. This condition is:

A. PID
B. Fitz-Hugh Curtis syndrome
C. Stein-Leventhal syndrome
D. Indistinct uterus
E. Meigs' syndrome

495. Pelvic ascites and right-sided pleural effusions can be associated with benign ovarian fibromas. This condition is:

A. Carcinoid syndrome
B. Turner's syndrome
C. Stein-Leventhal syndrome
D. Meigs' syndrome
E. Pseudosyndrome

This image applies to questions 496 and 497.

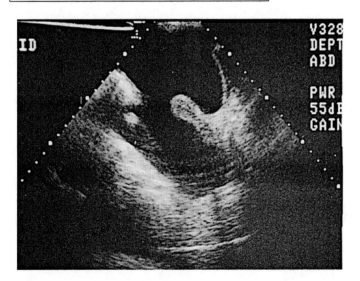

496. On bimanual pelvic examination, the clinician cannot palpate the uterus or ovaries. This image suggests:

A. Patient obesity
B. Atrophied organs
C. Bowel obstruction
D. Pelvic ascites

    E. Constipation

497. The arrow in this image is pointing to:

    A. Slice thickness artifact
    B. Reverberation
    C. Septation
    D. Debris
    E. Bowel

498. A patient who has taken oral contraceptives for more than 5 years is at increased risk for developing:

    A. Renal cancer
    B. Hepatic adenoma
    C. Heart disease
    D. Lung cancer
    E. Ectopic pregnancy

PART III

Patient Care Preparation/Technique

Review Charts
Explain Examinations
Supine Hypotensive Syndrome
Bioeffects
Infectious Disease Control
Scanning Techniques
Artifacts
Physical Principles

> **The following diagram applies to questions 499–502.**

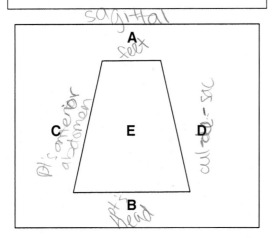

499. In transvaginal format, which letter would correspond to the patient's anterior abdomen when performing a sagittal scan?

A. A
B. B
C. C
D. D

E. E

500. In transvaginal format, which letter would correspond to the patient's cul-de-sac?

    A. A
    B. B
    C. C
    D. D
    E. E

501. In transvaginal format, which letter would be toward the patient's head if scanning in the sagittal plane?

    A. A
    B. B
    C. C
    D. D
    E. E

502. In transvaginal format, which letter would be toward the patient's feet if scanning in the sagittal plane?

    A. A
    B. B
    C. C
    D. D
    E. E

503. In the sagittal view, transvaginally, the bladder will be seen to fill:

    A. In the left lower corner of the image
    B. In the right lower corner of the image
 — C. In the left upper corner of the image
    D. In the right upper corner of the image
    E. In the middle anterior portion of the image

504. In the sagittal plane, transvaginally, the endometrial stripe is described as pointing toward the right lower corner of the image. The position of the uterus would be:

    A. Anteverted
    B. Anteflexed
    C. Retroverted
 — D. Retroflexed
    E. Inverted

505. A patient who is 38 weeks by good menstrual dates and 42 weeks by size is referred for sonographic estimation of fetal size. The patient cannot lie on her back without becoming restless, faint, and nauseated. She has what is called:

 —A. Supine hypotensive syndrome
    B. Hypertension

C. Hyperemesis gravidarum
D. Morning sickness
E. A virus

506. The best way to relieve the symptoms in the preceding patient would be to:

A. Give her some water and a cold cloth
B. Give her a Tums
C. Put her in the Trendelenburg's position
D. Give her antibiotics
E. Roll her onto her left side

507. The purpose of filling the urinary bladder prior to transabdominal ultrasonography includes all of the following EXCEPT:

A. Provides an acoustic window
B. Provides an internal cystic reference
C. Displaces bowel
D. Magnifies the pelvic organs
E. Flattens the uterine angle

508. For a transvaginal examination, the patient must be in the following position:

A. Lithotomy
B. Trendelenburg's
C. Prone
D. Decubitus
E. Reverse Trendelenburg's

509. The position of the fetus in this transverse drawing of a gravid uterus is:

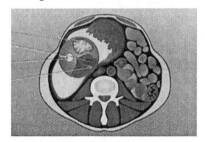

A. Breech presentation, longitudinal lie, spine on maternal right
B. Breech presentation, longitudinal lie, spine on maternal left
C. Cephalic presentation, longitudinal lie, spine on maternal left
D. Cephalic presentation, longitudinal lie, spine on maternal right.
E. Transverse oblique

Illustration reprinted with permission from Callen PW: The obstetrical ultrasound examination. In Callen PW (ed): *Ultrasonography in Obstetrics and Gynecology*, 4th edition. Philadelphia, WB Saunders, 2000, p 11.

510. The position of the fetus in this transverse drawing of a gravid uterus is:

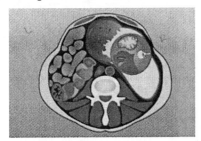

  A. Breech presentation, longitudinal lie, spine on maternal right
— B. Breech presentation, longitudinal lie, spine on maternal left
  C. Cephalic presentation, longitudinal lie, spine on maternal left
  D. Cephalic presentation, longitudinal lie, spine on maternal right.
  E. Transverse oblique

Illustration reprinted with permission from Callen PW: The obstetrical ultrasound examination. In Callen PW (ed): *Ultrasonography in Obstetrics and Gynecology*, 4ᵗʰ edition. Philadelphia, WB Saunders, 2000, p 11.

511. In this drawing the position of the fetus is:

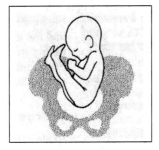

  A. Complete breech
  B. Full breech
— C. Frank breech
  D. Incomplete breech
  E. Footling breech

Illustration reprinted with permission from Callen PW: The obstetrical ultrasound examination. In Callen PW (ed): *Ultrasonography in Obstetrics and Gynecology*, 4ᵗʰ edition. Philadelphia, WB Saunders, 2000, p 13.

512. The position of the fetus in this longitudinal drawing of a gravid uterus is:

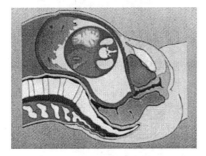

  A. Transverse lie with head on maternal right
— B. Transverse lie with head on maternal left
  C. Transverse lie with spine toward maternal feet

D. Cephalic presentation with spine on maternal right

E. Cephalic presentation with spine on maternal left

Illustration reprinted with permission from Callen PW: The obstetrical ultrasound examination. In Callen PW (ed): *Ultrasonography in Obstetrics and Gynecology*, 4ᵗʰ edition. Philadelphia, WB Saunders, 2000, p 12.

513. In this longitudinal drawing of a gravid uterus, the fetus is positioned:

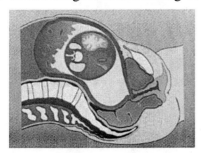

—A. Transverse with head on maternal right

B. Transverse with head on maternal left

C. Transverse with spine toward maternal head

D. Cephalic on maternal right

E. Cephalic on maternal left

Illustration reprinted with permission from Callen PW: The obstetrical ultrasound examination. In Callen PW (ed): *Ultrasonography in Obstetrics and Gynecology*, 4ᵗʰ edition. Philadelphia, WB Saunders, 2000, p 12.

514. Which of the following statements should NOT be written on the technical data sheet?

A. The uterus is normal in size and shape.

B. There is fluid noted in the cul-de-sac.

C. The left ovary is enlarged and hypoechoic.

D. There is no intrauterine pregnancy identified.

— E. There is an ectopic pregnancy identified in the right adnexa.

PART IV

Answers, Explanations & References

Obstetrics
Gynecology
Patient Care Preparation/Technique

OBSTETRICS

1.   C. Corpus luteal cyst

The corpus luteum cyst is a physiological cyst—it occurs normally as part of the menstrual cycle—that presents after ovulation. In the event of fertilization, the cyst produces progesterone necessary to maintain the pregnancy until the placenta develops and begins hormone production. These cysts usually resolve by 10–12 weeks.

2.   B. Rhombencephalon.

3.   A. Decidua basalis.

4.   B. 1 mm.

5.   D. 12 weeks

Physiological herniation is a normal developmental event that may be confused with true abdominal wall defects. The fetal small bowel develops so rapidly from gestational weeks 8 to 10 that the abdominal cavity cannot contain it. Fetal bowel protrudes into the base of the umbilical cord starting at 8 weeks gestation, peaking at 9 to 10 weeks gestation, and resolving by the 11th week of gestation as the fetal bowel retracts back into the intraabdominal cavity.

A case can be made for answer choice E, 14 weeks. Recent studies and evolving opinion offer support for this answer choice. Be aware of it. Nevertheless, the current editions of standard texts, general opinion, and long experience argue in favor of choosing 12 weeks as the answer on the ARDMS examination.

Studies indicate that normal physiological herniation is characterized by the following:

- *Physiological herniation will no longer be apparent once the crown rump length measures 45 mm or more.*

- *The base of the umbilical cord into which fetal bowel protrudes normally will not exceed 7 mm in diameter.*

- *Physiological herniation resolves by the 12th gestational week and should not be present thereafter. (But see note above.)*

Generally speaking, fetal physiologic bowel herniation should involute by 11 weeks but recent studies indicate that some cases do not involute until after 12 weeks. Despite the fact that pathologic defects of the fetal ventral abdominal wall can be observed at earlier gestational ages with high-resolution endovaginal sonography, distinction between physiologic bowel herniation and a pathological defect cannot always be made in the first trimester and must be followed carefully. The presence of any organ other than small bowel outside of the abdominal cavity represents—at any gestational age—a defect of the abdominal wall.

▷ Laing FC, Frates MC, Benson CB: Ultrasound evaluation during the first trimester of pregnancy. In Callen PW (ed): *Ultrasonography in Obstetrics and Gynecology*, 5th edition. Philadelphia, Saunders Elsevier, 2008, p 216.

▷ Bronshtein MB, Blazer S, Zimmer EZ: The gastrointestinal tract and abdominal wall. In Callen PW (ed): *Ultrasonography in Obstetrics and Gynecology*, 5th edition. Philadelphia, Saunders Elsevier, 2008, pp 587–634.

6.   E. 3600.

There are three different standards for measuring beta-hCG levels: (1) the Second International Standard, (2) the more recent International Reference Preparation (IRP) which uses values that are approximately double those of the 2nd International Standard (1.8 times the IS, to be exact), and most recently the Third International Standard, the values of which are similar to those of the IRP.

To identify a normal intrauterine pregnancy transabdominally, the IRP value should be $\geq$ 3600 mIU/ml and the 2nd International Standard $\geq$ 1800 mIU/ml. Transvaginally, IRP $\geq$ 2000 and 2nd International Standard $\geq$ 1000.

▷ Hickey J, Goldberg F: *Ultrasound Review of Obstetrics and Gynecology*. Philadelphia, Lippincott-Raven, 1996, p 68.

▷ Fleischer AC, Diamond MP, Cartwright PS: Transvaginal sonography of ectopic pregnancy. In ᐧ Fleischer AC, Manning FA, Jeanty P, et al (eds): *Sonography in Obstetrics and Gynecology: Principles and Practice*, 7th edition. McGraw Hill Professional, 2011, ch 2.

7.   C. Double decidual ring.

Identification of the double decidual ring is the sonographic criteria for determining whether there is a normal intrauterine gestational sac or just endometrial fluid surrounded by a decidualized endometrium.

8.   A. Retention of a dead conceptus for a prolonged period (e.g., 2 months).

These patients may or may not have bleeding.

9.   D. Fundal implantation.

10.   B. Hydatidiform mole.

In most cases, pregnancy-induced hypertension does not present until the second trimester. Preeclampsia in the first trimester is almost always pathognomonic of a molar pregnancy.

▷Beck WW Jr: Gestational trophoblastic neoplasia. In Beck WW Jr (ed): *Obstetrics and Gynecology, The National Medical Series for Independent Study*. Media, PA, Harwal Publishing, 1986, pp 173–175.

▷Pfeifer SM: *NMS Obstetrics and Gynecology (National Medical Series for Independent Study)*, 7th edition. Philadelphia, Lippincott Williams & Wilkins, 2011.

11.   E. Dilated cervix.

12.   B. An ectopic pregnancy with a normal intrauterine pregnancy.

If one can identify a normal intrauterine pregnancy, the likelihood of the patient having an ectopic pregnancy is negligible. However, fertility assistance has caused a slight increase in the incidence of heterotopic ectopic pregnancies.

13.   C. Yolk sac.

14.   E. 6 mm.

Large (greater than 6 mm), irregularly shaped, and calcified yolk sacs have all been found to correlate with early pregnancy failure.

▷ Laing FC, Frates MC, Benson CB: Ultrasound evaluation during the first trimester of pregnancy. In

Callen PW (ed): *Ultrasonography in Obstetrics and Gynecology*, 5th edition. Philadelphia, Saunders Elsevier, 2008, pp 208–209.

15. B. Methotrexate.

    Methotrexate is a folic acid antagonist used as an antineoplastic agent. It is also used in the treatment of psoriasis.

▷Miller BF, Keane CB: *Encyclopedia and Dictionary of Medicine, Nursing and Allied Health*, 7th edition. Philadelphia, WB Saunders, 2003, p 1121.

16. A. Leiomyoma.

17. C. Anteflexed.

18. B. Subchorionic hemorrhage.

19. C. Crown-rump length.

20. D. Yolk sac.

21. B. Normal early intrauterine pregnancy.

22. A. Interstitial.

    Interstitial implantation is very rare but very dangerous because rupture is accompanied by bleeding from uterine arteries. This type of ectopic pregnancy may be relatively asymptomatic and can progress without rupture up to 3–4 months.

▷ Levi CS, Lyons EA: The first trimester. In Rumack CM, Wilson SR, Charboneau JW, et al (eds): *Diagnostic Ultrasound*, 4th edition. St. Louis, Elsevier Mosby, 2010, pp 1072–1118.

▷Bain C, Burton K, McGavigan J, et al: *Gynaecology Illustrated*, 6th edition. New York, Churchill Livingstone, 2011, pp 320–323.

23. C. The amnion and yolk sac.

24. C. The sac is too small for a 10-week gestation suggesting incorrect dates.

    By eight weeks, the normal gestational sac should occupy one-half of the uterine cavity and show a yolk sac, embryo, and heart beat. By 10 weeks, the sac should have grown to fill the uterine cavity, and a well-defined fetus should be apparent.

25. A. Amnion.

26. E. Normal fetus.

The most common is the "complete" hydatidiform mole, which represents trophoblastic neoplasia without an embryo. With a "partial" mole, an abnormal embryo or fetus coexists with the mole.

▷Sohaey R: The first trimester. In Zwiebel WJ, Sohaey R: *Introduction to Ultrasound.* Philadelphia, WB Saunders, 1998, p 384.

▷Goldstein C, Hagen-Ansert SL: First trimester complications. In Hagen-Ansert SL (ed): *Textbook of Diagnostic Ultrasonography*, 7th edition. St. Louis, Mosby Elsevier, 2012, pp 1085–1086.

27. B. Crown-rump length.

28. E. 11 weeks.

The most accurate time to date a pregnancy by crown-rump length is in the first trimester, ideally at 10 weeks. By 11 weeks, spinal segmentation begins and gives the fetus the ability to curl, which may affect the accuracy of the measurement.

29. A. Vitelline duct.

The vitelline duct, also called the <u>omphalomesenteric duct</u>, is the structure that initially maintains a connection between the yolk sac and the embryo once they diverge from one another. The vitelline duct contains an artery and vein through which nutrients and blood elements are transported from the yolk sac to the embryo.

▷Laing FC, Frates MC, Benson CB: Ultrasound evaluation during the first trimester of pregnancy. In Callen PW (ed): *Ultrasonography in Obstetrics and Gynecology*, 5th edition. Philadelphia, Saunders Elsevier, 2008, pp 194–196.

30. B. Nuchal translucency.

31. C. It is a good indicator for possible chromosomal abnormalities.

An important finding of screening studies in high-risk pregnancies is that there is a strong correlation between chromosomal defects and both thickened fetal nuchal translucency—thickening of the nuchal soft tissues during the first trimester—and maternal age.

▷Nicolaides KH, Sebire NJ, Snijders RJM, et al: *The 11–14 Week Scan: The Diagnosis of Fetal Abnormalities.* New York, Parthenon Publishing, 2000, pp 6–36.

32. C. 8 weeks.

33. D. Early pregnancy failure.

34. D. A and B.

Shirodkar is the most complicated procedure, whereby the suture is almost completely buried beneath the cervical mucosa. It can be left in place for subsequent pregnancies if a cesarean is performed. McDonald is the simplest procedure, subjecting the cervix to less trauma and producing less blood loss than the Shirodkar procedure. It is a simple purse-string suture of the cervix.

▷Coney P: Operative obstetrics. In Beck WW Jr (ed): *Obstetrics and Gynecology, The National Medical Series for Independent Study.* New York, Harwal Publishing, 1986, pp 157–160.

▷Pfeifer SM: *NMS Obstetrics and Gynecology (National Medical Series for Independent Study),* 7th edition. Philadelphia, Lippincott Williams & Wilkins, 2011.

35. E. The ovary is the second most common site for ectopic pregnancy.

Approximately 97% of ectopic gestations occur in the fallopian tubes (93% ampullary; 4% isthmic). 2.5% of ectopic pregnancies are interstitial within the uterine cornua. Other ectopic implantation sites are nontubal and may uncommonly occur in the ovaries (0.5%), the cervix (0.12%), and the abdomen (0.03%)

▷Allen T, Cervantes F: Sonographic assessment of ectopic pregnancy. In Berman MC, Cohen HL (eds): *Diagnostic Medical Sonography, A Guide to Clinical Practice—Obstetrics and Gynecology,* 2nd edition. Philadelphia, Lippincott, 1997, pp 191–196.

36. C. 3 mm.

A nuchal translucency thickness exceeding 3 mm is associated with a significantly increased incidence of aneuploidy (abnormal karyotype). The abnormality most commonly associated with abnormal nuchal translucency—excessive thickening of the nuchal soft tissues during the first trimester—is trisomy 21.

▷Malone FD: First trimester screening for aneuploidy. In Callen PW (ed): *Ultrasonography in Obstetrics and Gynecology,* 5th edition. Philadelphia, Saunders Elsevier, 2008, pp 61–64, 66–69.

▷Saurbrei EE, Nguyen KT, Nolan RL, et al: *A Practical Guide to Ultrasound in Obstetrics and Gynecology.* Philadelphia, Lippincott-Raven, 1998, pp 140–141.

37. B. Within the atria of the lateral ventricles bilaterally.

38. D. Lateral ventricular atria.

The echogenic choroid plexus sits within the atria of the lateral ventricles and produces cerebrospinal fluid. Therefore this site will be the first at which fluid collects when there is obstruction or an overproduction of cerebrospinal fluid.

▷Toi A, Levine D: The fetal brain. In Rumack CM, Wilson SR, Charboneau JW, et al (eds): *Diagnostic Ultrasound*, 4th edition. St. Louis, Elsevier Mosby, 2010, pp 1197–1244.

39.   A. Cavum septum pellucidum.

40.   C. Cisterna magna.

41.   C. 1 cm in the largest dimension transversely.

42.   B. Thalami.

43.   B. Choroid plexus.

44.   C. Posterior fossa.

45.   C. 4th ventricle.

46.   C. Cerebellum.

47.   D. Three ossification centers, two posterior and one anterior, with the two posterior centers pointing toward each other.

48.   D. Pedicles and lamina.

▷Sauerbrei E: The fetal spine. In Rumack CM, Wilson SR, Charboneau JW, et al (eds): *Diagnostic Ultrasound*, 4th edition. St. Louis, Elsevier Mosby, 2010, pp 1245–1272.

49.   C. Centrum.

▷ Sauerbrei E: The fetal spine. In Rumack CM, Wilson SR, Charboneau JW, et al (eds): *Diagnostic Ultrasound*, 4th edition. St. Louis, Elsevier Mosby, 2010, pp 1245–1272.

50.   A. Laminae.

▷ Sauerbrei E: The fetal spine. In Rumack CM, Wilson SR, Charboneau JW, et al (eds): *Diagnostic Ultrasound*, 4th edition. St. Louis, Elsevier Mosby, 2010, pp 1245–1272.

51.   D. Spinous process.

▷ Sauerbrei E: The fetal spine. In Rumack CM, Wilson SR, Charboneau JW, et al (eds): *Diagnostic Ultrasound*, 4th edition. St. Louis, Elsevier Mosby, 2010, pp 1245–1272.

52.   C. M-mode.

53. B. Left atrium

54. D. One-third of the chest cavity pointing toward the left side of the fetus.

As the fetus develops, the circumference of its heart remains approximately one-half the circumference of the thorax. The apex of the fetal heart tilts toward the left side of the thoracic cavity. The fetal heart is forced into a position more horizontal than it is postnatally by the fetal diaphragm, which is situated relatively high in the chest because of the fetus's large liver and uninflated lungs.

▷Yoo SJ, Jaeggi E: Ultrasound evaluation of the fetal heart. In Callen PW (ed): *Ultrasonography in Obstetrics and Gynecology*, 5th edition. Philadelphia, Saunders Elsevier, 2008, 511–586.

55. D. A and C.

▷Cyr DR, Gentheroth WG, et al: Fetal echocardiography. In Berman MC, Cohen HL (eds): *Diagnostic Medical Sonography, A Guide to Clinical Practice—Obstetrics and Gynecology*, 2nd edition. Philadelphia, Lippincott, 1997, pp 321–326.

▷Hagen-Ansert SL: Fetal echocardiography: beyond the four chambers. In Hagen-Ansert SL (ed): *Textbook of Diagnostic Ultrasonography*, 7th edition. St. Louis, Mosby Elsevier, 2012, pp 822–824.

56. C. Right ventricle.

57. C. Tricuspid valve.

58. D. Foramen ovale.

59. D. Transverse aorta.

60. D. 45° to the left of midline.

In the normal fetus the axis of the ventricular septum and anatomic midline is about 45°. Significant displacement to the right or left of this 45° angle may indicate heart disease.

▷ Yoo SJ, Jaeggi E: Ultrasound evaluation of the fetal heart. In Callen PW (ed): *Ultrasonography in Obstetrics and Gynecology*, 5th edition. Philadelphia, Saunders Elsevier, 2008, 511–586.

61. C. Pulmonary artery and ascending aorta.

62. B. LVOT.

63. C. Chordae tendineae/papillary muscle.

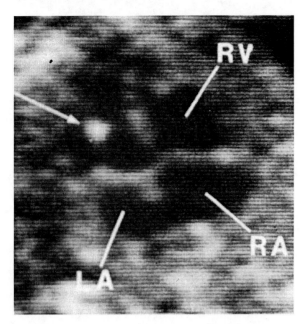

An echogenic focus may be seen in the right as well as the left ventricles. These usually correspond to the moderator band in the right ventricle and/or the papillary muscle or chordae tendineae in either ventricle. See example above.

▷Stamm E, Drose J: The fetal heart. In Rumack CM, Wilson SR, Charboneau JW, et al (eds): *Diagnostic Ultrasound*, 4th edition. St. Louis, Elsevier Mosby, 2010, pp 1294–1326.

64.   B. Right atrium.

65.   A. Right ventricle.

66.   E. Aorta.

67.   C. Right ventricular outflow tract.

68.   C. Ascending aorta.

69.   D. Descending aorta.

70.   E. Diaphragm.

71.   A. Left atrium.

72.   E. Coronal.

      Actually, both coronal and parasagittal views often allow one to image the diaphragm.

73.   B. True transverse view at the level of the fetal 4-chamber heart.

74.   D. Aortic arch.

75.   A. Artifact.

Shadowing in the far field makes the contralateral lung less echogenic. The echogenicity of the lungs should <u>never</u> be used to determine fetal lung maturity. Tracheal atresia results in bilaterally increased echogenicity.

76.   C. Esophageal atresia.

Visualization of the fluid-filled fetal stomach is an important part of the basic scan. The fetal stomach should be seen filled with fluid during the course of an exam.

> ▷Abbott J: The fetal abdominal wall and gastrointestinal tract. In Rumack CM, Wilson SR, Charboneau JW, et al (eds): *Diagnostic Ultrasound*, 4th edition. St. Louis, Elsevier Mosby, 2010, pp 1327–1354.

77.   D. Gallbladder.

78.   B. The presence and evaluation of urine in the fetal bladder and amniotic fluid by approximately 13 weeks gestation.

After 12–13 weeks gestation the amniotic fluid volume and, obviously, fluid in the fetal bladder are almost entirely due to functioning kidneys. Prior to this time, amniotic fluid may be a result of transudation from the placenta and membranes.

> ▷ Saurbrei EE, Nguyen KT, Nolan RL, et al: *A Practical Guide to Ultrasound in Obstetrics and Gynecology*. Philadelphia, Lippincott-Raven, 1998, pp 325–330.

> ▷Spitz JL: Sonography of the second and third trimesters. In Hagen-Ansert SL (ed): *Textbook of Diagnostic Ultrasonography*, 7th edition. St. Louis, Mosby Elsevier, 2012, pp 1130–1132.

79.   C. Adjacent to the fetal spine bilaterally.

80.   C. 30–45 minutes.

Although bladder refill times vary, answer C is the best choice. A, B, D, and E are all either too short or too long as an approximation of average bladder refill time.

> ▷Fong KW, Robertson J, Maxwell CV: The fetal urogenital tract. In Rumack CM, Wilson SR, Charboneau JW, et al (eds): *Diagnostic Ultrasound*, 4th edition. St. Louis, Elsevier Mosby, 2010, pp 1353–1388.

> ▷Avni FE, Maugey-Laulom B, Cassart M, et al: The fetal genitourinary tract. In Callen PW (ed): *Ultrasonography in Obstetrics and Gynecology*, 5th edition. Philadelphia, Saunders Elsevier, 2008, p 642.

81.   D. Adrenal gland.

82. B. Posterior urethral valves.

Posterior urethral valves, which obstruct the posterior urethra, are the most common cause of bladder outlet obstruction in the male fetus. The sonographic presentation includes a persistent and oftentimes profoundly dilated bladder or thickened bladder walls. Distention of the posterior urethra is sometimes visualized, and moderate to severe oligohydramnios may be present when the obstruction affects the fetus's ability to void into the amniotic sac, as is often the case. Although obstruction of the bladder outlet mainly affects the male fetus, the female fetus also may suffer from urethral obstruction secondary to a number of pathologies. In the female, the most common cause of urethral obstruction is cloacal malformation or urethral atresia.

▷ Avni FE, Maugey-Laulom B, Cassart M, et al: The fetal genitourinary tract. In Callen PW (ed): *Ultrasonography in Obstetrics and Gynecology*, 5th edition. Philadelphia, Saunders Elsevier, 2008, p 649.

83. C. 16 weeks gestation.

84. B. Female.

85. B. Iliac bones.

86. C. Abdominal circumference.

87. E. Supine hypotensive syndrome.

88. E. All of the above.

89. D. Amniocentesis.

90. D. Fetal anatomy.

91. E. All of the above.

92. E. A and C.

▷Glanc P, Chitayat D, Unger S: The fetal musculoskeletal system. In Rumack CM, Wilson SR, Charboneau JW, et al (eds): *Diagnostic Ultrasound*, 4th edition. St. Louis, Elsevier Mosby, 2010, pp 1389–1423.

93. C. Shows a good position for identifying club foot.

94. C. Vertex.

95.   B. Transverse fetal head right.

96.   C. Vasa previa.

A vasa previa denotes umbilical vessels that are not supported by normal cord structures that cross the internal cervical os. This condition exists when there is either a succenturiate lobe of the placenta or a velamentous insertion of the umbilical cord. In both cases umbilical vessels might travel in the membranes across the internal os to reach the insertion site into the placenta.

97.   C. 37th week of gestation.

98.   D. Ascending aorta.

99.   A. Cleft lip.

100. A. Normal kidney.

101. E. B and C.

102. B. Excessive Wharton's jelly.

103. A. Produces alphafetoprotein.

Alphafetoprotein is produced by the fetal liver and GI tract and excreted into the amniotic fluid. By diffusion across the placenta, it makes its way into the maternal bloodstream. Therefore the level of maternal serum alphafetoprotein (MSAFP) can be measured in the maternal blood.

104. C. Succenturiate.

Focal failure of the chorion villi, not in contact with the deciduas basalis, to atrophy may result in development of a mass of placental tissue separate from the main body of the placenta but connected by common vessels. This tissue is referred to as a succenturiate, accessory, or supernumerary placenta.

▷Feldstein VA, Harris RD, Machin GA: Ultrasound evaluation of the placenta and umbilical cord. In Callen PW (ed): *Ultrasonography in Obstetrics and Gynecology*, 5th edition. Philadelphia, Saunders Elsevier, 2008, p 724.

105. D. 2 cm.

The low-lying placenta may be difficult to distinguish from a placenta previa. A placenta is usually described as low-lying when the lower margin is < 2 cm from the internal cervical os.

▷Nolan RL: The placenta, membranes, umbilical cord, and amniotic fluid. In Saurbrei EE, Nguyen KT, Nolan RL, et al (eds): *A Practical Guide to*

Ultrasound in Obstetrics and Gynecology, 2nd edition. Philadelphia, Lippincott-Raven, 1998, pp 445–450.

▷Foy P: The placenta. In Hagen-Ansert SL (ed): *Textbook of Diagnostic Ultrasonography*, 7th edition. St. Louis, Mosby Elsevier, 2012, pp 1229–1230.

106. C. Anterior marginal.

107. A. Retroplacental space.

108. E. Normal retroplacental space.

109. B. Posterior.

110. A. Placenta accreta.

Placenta accreta is detected ultrasonographically through analysis of the retroplacental complex. The ultrasound criteria for identifying placenta accreta are:

- *Loss of normal hypoechoic retroplacental myometrial zone (most common but least specific sign), which should measure 1 to 2 cm but which in placenta accreta is absent or significantly thinned to 2 mm or less*
- *Loss of normal venous Doppler flow at site*
- *Thinning of the myometrium adjacent to the placenta*
- *Loss of the hyperechoic uterine serosal boundary*
- *Nodular projection of placental tissue beyond the serosal margin (least common but most specific sign)*
- *Numerous intraparenchymal lacunar vascular spaces (venous lakes)*

▷ Nolan RL: The placenta, membranes, umbilical cord, and amniotic fluid. In Saurbrei EE, Nguyen KT, Nolan RL, et al (eds): *A Practical Guide to Ultrasound in Obstetrics and Gynecology*, 2nd edition. Philadelphia, Lippincott-Raven, 1998, p 444.

▷ Feldstein VA, Harris RD, Machin GA: Ultrasound evaluation of the placenta and umbilical cord. In Callen PW (ed): *Ultrasonography in Obstetrics and Gynecology*, 5th edition. Philadelphia, Saunders Elsevier, 2008, pp 737–742.

111. D. Hypertension.

Small placentas may be associated with:

- *IUGR*
- *Toxemia of pregnancy*
- *Maternal hypertension*
- *Chromosomal abnormality*

- *Severe maternal diabetes*
- *Intrauterine infection*

The conditions most commonly associated with thick placenta are:

- *Maternal diabetes mellitus*
- *Hydrops fetalis (immune/nonimmune)*
- *Infection*
- *Trisomy/triploidy*
- *Anemia*
- *Hydatidiform mole*
- *Intraplacental hemorrhage*
- *Villitis*
- *Beckwith-Wiedemann syndrome*

▷Nolan RL: *A Practical Guide to Ultrasound in Obstetrics and Gynecology*, 2nd edition. Philadelphia, Lippincott-Raven, 1998, p 441.

▷ Feldstein VA, Harris RD, Machin GA: Ultrasound evaluation of the placenta and umbilical cord. In Callen PW (ed): *Ultrasonography in Obstetrics and Gynecology*, 5th edition. Philadelphia, Saunders Elsevier, 2008, pp 721–744.

112. C. 4 cm.

The thickness of a full-term placenta rarely exceeds 4 cm. As a general rule, the thickness of a placenta, measured in millimeters, should approximate the gestational age of the fetus, measured in weeks, plus or minus 10 mm.

▷ Feldstein VA, Harris RD, Machin GA: Ultrasound evaluation of the placenta and umbilical cord. In Callen PW (ed): *Ultrasonography in Obstetrics and Gynecology*, 5th edition. Philadelphia, Saunders Elsevier, 2008, pp 721–744.

113. B. A grade III placenta indicates fetal lung maturity.

Placentas are similar to humans. Like us, placentas age at different rates. The rate at which the placenta ages is affected by maternal conditions and practices. Smokers' placentas tend to age more rapidly, for instance, while diabetics often show a grade 0 placenta at term. As a general rule, one should not see a grade III placenta before 35–37 weeks because this would suggest that the placenta has reached an advanced age. The only sure way to determine fetal lung maturity is by checking the L/S (lecithin/sphingomyelin) ratio through amniocentesis.

▷ Callen PW (ed): *Ultrasonography in Obstetrics and Gynecology*, 5th edition. Philadelphia, Saunders Elsevier, 2008, pp 224, 494, 725.

114. D. Chorioangioma.

Chorioangiomas are benign vascular tumors of the placenta. They rarely get large enough to identify sonographically. Large ones should be monitored because they can cause IUGR, hydrops, and placental abruption.

115. D. Grade III.

116. B. Superior to the fetal bladder.

117. D. Cord insertion.

118. B. Two umbilical arteries.

Upon entering the fetal abdomen just superior to the fetal bladder, the two umbilical arteries within the cord split and can be seen on either side of the fetal bladder.

119. C. Placental abruption.

120. A. Total placenta previa.

121. C. Cerebral thalami.

122. B. 61%.

Cephalic index (CI, expressed as %) = BPD/OFD x 100
Normal cephalic index range = 70–85%
Low CI = dolichocephaly
High CI = brachycephaly

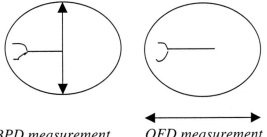

BPD measurement   *OFD measurement*

BPD = biparietal diameter, OFD = occipital frontal diameter (also FOD, fronto-occipital diameter).

▷Hickey J, Goldberg F: *Ultrasound Review of Obstetrics and Gynecology.* Philadelphia, Lippincott-Raven, 1996, p 155.

▷DuBose TJ, Hagen-Ansert SL: Obstetric measurements and gestational age. In Hagen-Ansert

SL (ed): *Textbook of Diagnostic Ultrasonography*, 7th
edition. St. Louis, Mosby Elsevier, 2012, p 1150.

123. A. Dolichocephaly.

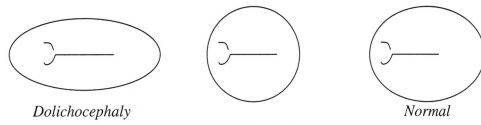

Dolichocephaly   Normal

Brachycephaly

Dolichocephaly is a head shape that is too long and narrow. This shape will cause the BPD to measure much smaller in weeks when compared with the circumference and femur length measurements. Brachycephaly is an abnormally short head length.

124. B. Crown-rump length at 10 weeks.

125. D. 30 weeks.

▷ Galan HL, Pandipati S, Filly RA: Ultrasound
evaluation of fetal biometry and normal and abnormal
fetal growth. In Callen PW (ed): *Ultrasonography in
Obstetrics and Gynecology*, 5th edition. Philadelphia,
Saunders Elsevier, 2008, pp 225–265.

126. C. 30 weeks.

127. B. Leading edge.

This method of caliper placement was established because the artifactual thickening of the most posterior skull table makes it difficult to know precisely where the middle or true edge of the skull is. The leading edge technique eliminates the problem and makes measurements more reliably reproducible.

128. D. Amniocentesis.

129. C. Head shape.

130. A. Naegele's rule.

131. C. Quickening.

Quickening is the sensation of fetal movement. Between the 16th and 20th weeks after the last menstrual period, a woman begins to feel movement in the lower abdomen described as fluttering or gas bubbles.

▷Miller BF, Keane CB, O'Toole MT: *Encyclopedia
and Dictionary of Medicine, Nursing and Allied*

Health, 7th edition. Philadelphia, WB Saunders, 2005, p 1491.

▷Beck WW: *Obstetrics and Gynecology: The National Medical Series for Independent Study.* Media, PA, Harwal Publishing, 1986, p 25.

▷Pfeifer SM: *NMS Obstetrics and Gynecology (National Medical Series for Independent Study)*, 7th edition. Philadelphia, Lippincott Williams & Wilkins, 2011.

132. A. 1 mm.

Monitoring sac growth can be reliable up to 10 weeks menstrual age, at which time the sac should fill the uterine cavity. Sac measurements are obtained by calculating the mean sac diameter. The dimensions of the sac are measured in long axis, transverse, and anterior-posterior views. The average of these three measurements is the <u>mean sac diameter</u> (MSD). Care should be taken not to include the decidual echoes in the measurements. Calipers are placed on the inner surfaces to measure the inside diameter.

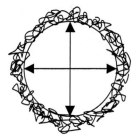

133. C. 3.

134. B. 2 weeks.

135. D. BPD/OFD x 100.

136. E. Nuchal skin fold.

Nuchal skin fold thickening has been associated with chromosomal abnormalities, particularly Down's syndrome. The thickened fold can be seen at the level of the BPD/HC. The thickness should not measure more than 5 mm; however, this criteria is not reliable after 24 weeks.

137. A. Angle of asynclitism.

The angle of asynclitism refers to the tilt of the fetal head in utero. By viewing the fetal head longitudinally and evaluating the angle of tilt, one can determine the necessary degree of angulation of the sound beam when attempting to obtain BPD/HC measurements coronally. The sound beam should be perpendicular to the angle of the fetal head.

138. C. Clavicle.

139. E. B and D.

The ideal landmark for localizing the correct level at which abdominal circumference can be correctly measured is the fetal umbilical vein where it can be seen turning into the portal vein. It will have the characteristic "hockey stick" appearance. Unfortunately, fetal position sometimes precludes that perfect image, in which case other fetal anatomical structures must be identified. The fetal adrenal glands, stomach, and gallbladder are all seen at the same level as the umbilical vein, and therefore the abdominal circumference can be measured where these organs are identified.

140. B. It is considered more accurate than the biparietal diameter measurement.

Both biparietal diameter (BPD) and head circumference (HC) should be measured at the level of the cerebral thalami. Unlike head circumference, the biparietal diameter can be affected by head shape. BPD measurements are therefore considered less reliable than HC measurements. For this reason, the cephalic index (CI) should always be evaluated. The shape of the fetal head can be affected by such things as breech presentation, ruptured membranes, and multiple gestations.

▷ Galan HL, Pandipati S, Filly RA: Ultrasound evaluation of fetal biometry and normal and abnormal fetal growth. In Callen PW (ed): *Ultrasonography in Obstetrics and Gynecology*, 5th edition. Philadelphia, Saunders Elsevier, 2008, pp 225–265.

141. B. Calculates fetal heart rate according to fetal activity.

Nonstress test (NST)—or fetal activity test (FAT)—is a noninvasive test of fetal activity that correlates with fetal well being. Fetal heart acceleration is observed during fetal movement. An external fetal monitor is used to record the fetal heart rate (FHR), and the mother participates by indicating fetal movements. A reactive test reveals 3 or more fetal movements over 30 minutes with fetal heart acceleration of at least 15 beats' amplitude of 15 seconds' duration.

▷Beck WW: *Obstetrics and Gynecology: The National Medical Series for Independent Study.* Media, PA, Harwal Publishing, 1986, p 57.

▷Pfeifer SM: *NMS Obstetrics and Gynecology (National Medical Series for Independent Study)*, 7th edition. Philadelphia, Lippincott Williams & Wilkins, 2011.

142. E. Cleft defects.

143. A. Monozygotic.

144. B. Monozygotic twins share the same amniotic sac.

     Monozygotic twins occur as the result of division of one fertilized ovum during the period after fertilization. Depending on the time of division, chorionicity and amnionicity can be di or mono. Only 1–2% of monozygotic twins will be monoamniotic.

     ▷Jaffe R, Abramowicz JS: *Manual of Obstetric and Gynecologic Ultrasound.* Philadelphia, Lippincott-Raven, 1997, pp 199–201.

     ▷Mitchell C, Trampe B: Sonography and high-risk pregnancy. In Hagen-Ansert SL (ed): *Textbook of Diagnostic Ultrasonography*, 7th edition. St. Louis, Mosby Elsevier, 2012, pp 1182–1185.

145. D. Caudal regression syndrome.

146. D. Trisomy 21.

     Approximately 20% of fetuses with trisomy 21 are found in women whose MSAFP level is low after adjustment for age. When the MSAFP level is low the risk of trisomy is significant enough to warrant amniocentesis for karyotyping.

     ▷ Norton ME: Genetics and prenatal diagnosis. In Callen PW (ed): *Ultrasonography in Obstetrics and Gynecology*, 5th edition. Philadelphia, Saunders Elsevier, 2008, p 45.

147. A. Ventricular measurements are consistent throughout pregnancy.

148. B. Thanatophoric dwarfism.

149. D. Vein of Galen aneurysm.

150. A. It is compatible with life and carries a good prognosis.

     Holoprosencephaly: alobar (most severe), semilobar, and lobar (least severe). The prognosis is dismal for both alobar and semilobar, and variable for the lobar form.

     ▷Johnson PT, Kurtz AB: *Case Review Obstetric and Gynecologic Ultrasound.* Mosby, St. Louis, 2001, pp 35–36.

     ▷Reuter K, Babagbemi TK: *Obstetric and Gynecologic Ultrasound: Case Review Series.* St. Louis, Mosby, 2006.

151. C. FL/AC.

152. E. GI tract obstruction.

153. D. A and B.

154. A. Transposition of the great vessels.

The four-chamber view often overlooks small or subtle intracardiac defects. In addition, the four-chamber view cannot identify the aorta and pulmonary arteries.

▷Middleton WD, Kurtz AB, Hertzberg BS:
Ultrasound: The Requisites, 2nd edition. St. Louis,
Mosby, 2004, pp 416–419.

155. C. Ventricular.

Imaging the atria of the ventricles is part of the basic guidelines; however, measuring them is currently optional. If measurements are performed, one should measure perpendicularly across the thickest portion of the choroid plexus.

156. B. Asynclitism.

157. B. Anencephaly.

158. C. Lens of the eye.

159. D. Pleural effusions.

160. D. Cystic hygroma.

161. A. Turner's.

162. D. Twins.

163. B. Lecithin/sphingomyelin ratio.

164. E. After delivery.

The puerperium is the period from termination of labor to complete involution of the uterus, a process that normally takes from 6 to 8 weeks.

165. E. 4 weeks.

166. D. Coexistent mole and live fetus.

167. C. Myometrial contraction.

168. E. A contraction.

169. B. There is an increased incidence if the father was a twin.

Dizygotic twins result from multiple ovulations that can be induced by gonadotropins or drugs such as clomiphene (commonly used in patients with

infertility). Therefore, fetal number is determined by the female while fetal sex is determined by the male.

▷Standring S (ed): *Gray's Anatomy*, 40th edition. New York, Churchill-Livingstone Elsevier, 2008, p 178.

170. E. 30 weeks.

171. D. Erythroblastosis fetalis.

Erythroblastosis fetalis (RH incompatibility)–a form of fetal anemia in which the fetal red cells are destroyed by contact with a maternal antibody produced in response to a previous fetus. Severe fetal heart failure results.

▷Sanders RC: *Clinical Sonography: A Practical Guide*, 3rd edition. Philadelphia, Lippincott, 1998, p 124.

▷Sanders RC: *Clinical Sonography: A Practical Guide*, 4th edition. Philadelphia, Lippincott, 2006.

172. A. Macrosomia.

173. B. Rhogam.

Rhogam is not necessary until after the first pregnancy and it is administered after delivery. As a precautionary measure, the patient will be given rhogam during future pregnancies usually at 28 and 32 weeks.

174. C. Packed red blood cells are introduced into the umbilical vein.

175. B. Cesarean section.

176. C. Pelvicaliectasis, during pregnancy, is most often observed on the left side.

Pelvicaliectasis and hydroureter are usually regarded as physiologic processes during pregnancy. The cause is postulated to be the result of a combination of extrinsic compression and hormonal effect. The right side is affected 90% of the time and the left side in approximately 67% of patients.

▷Sauerbrei EE, Nguyen KT, Nolan RL: *A Practical Guide to Ultrasound in Obstetrics and Gynecology*, 2nd edition. Philadelphia, Lippincott-Raven, 1998, pp 528–529.

177. B. Chorioadenoma destruens.

Although this type of mole is considered malignant because of its invasive nature, it is relatively harmless.

178. A. Cerclage.

179. C. Treat an incompetent cervix.

180. B. 6–8 weeks.

181. D. Uterine atony.

Uterine contractions after delivery are mostly responsible for squeezing off small bleeding vessels. If the uterus is unable to adequately contract, bleeding will persist. This is a complication when the uterus becomes too large due to multiple gestations, macrosomia, and gross polyhydramnios.

182. B. Acardiac twin.

Acardiac twins are rare and occur in 1 in 34,600 pregnancies. It is the most extreme manifestation of the twin transfusion syndrome and usually has a large arterial-to-arterial anastomosis. The pump donor twin supplies blood to itself and to the acardiac/recipient/perfused twin. The reversal of blood flow to the recipient acardiac twin is called twin reversed arterial perfusion pathophysiology (TRAP).

▷Sauerbrei EE, Nguyen KT, Nolan RL: *A Practical Guide to Ultrasound in Obstetrics and Gynecology*, 2nd edition. Philadelphia, Lippincott-Raven, 1998, pp 426–427.

▷Egan JFX, Borgida AF: Ultrasound evaluation of multiple pregnancies. In Callen PW (ed): *Ultrasonography in Obstetrics and Gynecology*, 5th edition. Philadelphia, Saunders Elsevier, 2008, pp 286–288.

183. A. Macrosomic.

184. E. TORCH.

185. D. Diuretics.

Diuretics can reduce renal perfusion and uteroplacental perfusion in a situation where there is already constricted intravascular volume.

▷Beck WW: *Obstetrics and Gynecology: The National Medical Series for Independent Study.* Media, PA, Harwal Publishing, 1986, p 64.

▷Pfeifer SM: *NMS Obstetrics and Gynecology (National Medical Series for Independent Study)*, 7th edition. Philadelphia, Lippincott Williams & Wilkins, 2011.

186. C. Fetal eye movement.

187. E. Pregnancy induced hypertension.

188. D. 24 cm.

Three values are used to calculate the amniotic index. They are:

(1)
< 8 cm = oligo
> 24 cm = poly
(Tends to overestimate oligohydramnios.)

(2)
< 5 cm = oligo
> 20 cm = poly

(3)
13 cm ± 10 which equates to
< 3 cm = oligo
> 23 cm = poly
(Tends to underestimate oligohydramnios.)

189. B. Intrauterine growth restriction.

The word <u>DRIP</u> can help you remember the causes for oligohydramnios. D = demise, R = renal anomalies, I = IUGR, and P = PROM.

190. E. Provides nourishment.

▷Jaffe R, Abramowicz JS: *Manual of Obstetric & Gynecologic Ultrasound.* Philadelphia, Lippincott-Raven, 1997, pp 188–189.

▷Robert M: Amniotic fluid, fetal membranes, and fetal hydrops. In Hagen-Ansert SL (ed): *Textbook of Diagnostic Ultrasonography,* 7th edition. St. Louis, Mosby Elsevier, 2012, p 1250.

191. A. Amniotic fluid index.

192. C. Meconium.

Fetuses do not normally expel meconium unless they are in distress. Meconium refers to fetal bowel contents and will present as flecks of green colored spinach-like material floating within the amniotic fluid. Vernix is the shedding of skin and hair that occurs naturally toward the end of pregnancy. These flecks will be whitish in color or show short fine strands of hair.

193. C. Fetal kidneys.

Before the fetal kidneys actually begin to function, amniotic fluid is secreted by the amnion. Between 12–15 weeks, fetal kidneys begin functioning to produce amniotic fluid.

194. C. Multiples of the median (MoM).

▷ Norton ME: Genetics and prenatal diagnosis. In Callen PW (ed): *Ultrasonography in Obstetrics and Gynecology*, 5th edition. Philadelphia, Saunders Elsevier, 2008, p 43.

195. E. A, C, and D.

Triple marker screening measures AFP, uE3, and hCG to determine the risk of Down's syndrome. Triple marker screening is also called the triple test. It is more sensitive than MSAFP measurements alone, with detection rates of from 58% to 91% and a false-positive rate of 5% to 6%.

▷ Norton ME: Genetics and prenatal diagnosis. In Callen PW (ed): *Ultrasound in Obstetrics and Gynecology*, 5th edition. Philadelphia, Saunders Elsevier, 2008, pp 45–46.

▷ Levine D: Overview of obstetric imaging. In Rumack CM, Wilson SR, Charboneau JW, et al (eds): *Diagnostic Ultrasound*, 4th edition. St. Louis, Elsevier Mosby, 2010, pp 1040–1060.

196. C. Hydatidiform mole.

Because there is no fetus in a complete molar pregnancy, little or no AFP is produced, thereby decreasing the MSAFP.

▷ Norton ME: Genetics and prenatal diagnosis. In Callen PW (ed): *Ultrasonography in Obstetrics and Gynecology*, 5th edition. Philadelphia, Saunders Elsevier, 2008, pp 42–45.

197. D. Gastrointestinal obstruction.

▷Wald NJ, Cuckle HS: Complementary use of biochemical tests and ultrasonography for detection of neural tube defects and down's syndrome: screening. In Chervenak FA, Isaacson GC, Campbell S (eds): *Ultrasound in Obstetrics and Gynecology*, volume 2. Boston, Little, Brown, 1993, pp 1135–1142.

▷Henningsen CG: Prenatal diagnosis of congenital anomalies. In Hagen-Ansert SL (ed): *Textbook of Diagnostic Ultrasonography*, 7th edition. St. Louis, Mosby Elsevier, 2012, p 1196.

198. A. Spina bifida.

▷Wald NJ, Cuckle HS: Complementary use of biochemical tests and ultrasonography for detection of neural tube defects and down's syndrome: screening. In Chervenak FA, Isaacson GC, Campbell S (eds): *Ultrasound in Obstetrics and Gynecology*, volume 2. Boston, Little, Brown, 1993, pp 1135–1142.

▷Norton M: Genetics and prenatal diagnosis. In Callen PW (ed): *Ultrasound in Obstetrics and Gynecology*, 5th edition. Philadelphia, Saunders Elsevier, 2008, p 44.

199. D. Amniocentesis sometimes unnecessary for prenatal diagnosis.

▷Benacherraf B: *Ultrasound of Fetal Syndromes*, 2nd edition. New York, Churchill Livingston, 2007.

200. E. A and C.

▷ Wladimiroff JW, Cohen-Overbeek TE, Laudy JAM: Ultrasound evaluation of the fetal thorax. In Callen PW (ed): *Ultrasound in Obstetrics and Gynecology*, 5th edition. Philadelphia, Saunders Elsevier, 2008, pp 493–508.

201. C. PUBS (percutaneous umbilical blood sampling).

▷Solish G: Amniocentesis and chorionic villus sampling. In Berman MC, Cohen HL: *Diagnostic Medical Sonography: A Guide to Clinical Practice: Obstetrics and Gynecology*, 2nd edition. Philadelphia, Lippincott, 1997, pp 579–589.

202. B. 15–16 weeks.

▷Solish G: Amniocentesis and chorionic villus sampling. In Berman MC, Cohen HL: *Diagnostic Medical Sonography: A Guide to Clinical Practice: Obstetrics and Gynecology*, 2nd edition. Philadelphia, Lippincott, 1997, pp 579–589.

203. E. The transabdominal technique is most commonly used.

▷Solish G: Amniocentesis and chorionic villus sampling. In Berman MC, Cohen HL: *Diagnostic Medical Sonography: A Guide to Clinical Practice: Obstetrics and Gynecology*, 2nd edition. Philadelphia, Lippincott, 1997, pp 579–589.

▷Tempkin BB, Bizjak PM: The female pelvis. In Curry RA, Tempkin BB (eds): *Sonography: Introduction to Normal Structure and Function*, 3rd edition. Philadelphia, Elsevier Saunders, 2011, p 358.

204. C. 10–13 weeks.

▷Solish G: Amniocentesis and chorionic villus sampling. In Berman MC, Cohen HL: *Diagnostic Medical Sonography: A Guide to Clinical Practice: Obstetrics and Gynecology*, 2nd edition. Philadelphia, Lippincott, 1997, pp 579–589.

▷Hamar B: Ultrasound-guided invasive fetal procedures. In Rumack CM, Wilson SR, Charboneau JW, et al (eds): *Diagnostic Ultrasound*, 4th edition. St. Louis, Elsevier Mosby, 2010, p 1545.

205. B. Autosomal dominant.

▷Goljan E: *Most Commons In Medicine.*
Philadelphia, WB Saunders, 2000, pp 51–56.

206. B. The father must have the disease in order to pass it on to his children.

X-linked genes in the XY male are present in a single dose with no partner gene. Hence, a single copy of the mutant gene on the X chromosome will express a full recessive disorder. The probability of an XX female having a pair of such X-linked recessive genes and expressing the same disorder as the XY male is very low. The following generalization applies to this pattern of inheritance: with rare exceptions, only males are affected.

▷Jones KL: *Smith's Recognizable Patterns of Human Malformation*, 6th edition. Philadelphia, Saunders Elsevier, 2006.

▷Goljan E: *Most Commons In Medicine.*
Philadelphia, WB Saunders, 2000, pp 51–56.

207. C. Failure of mother to feel fetal movement is diagnostic.

▷Callen PW: The obstetric ultrasound examination. In Callen PW (ed): *Ultrasonography in Obstetrics and Gynecology*, 5th edition. Philadelphia, Saunders Elsevier, 2008, p 14.

208. C. Calcified fetus.

209. E. Unknown cause.

Although the causes of fetal death can vary, depending on the part of the world the death occurs and the life style associated with that part of the world, the most common cause of death remains to be unknown.

▷Nolan RL: The maternal abdomen and pelvis in pregnancy. In Sauerbrei, Nguyen KT, Nolan RL (eds): *A Practical Guide to Ultrasound in Obstetrics and Gynecology*, 2nd edition. Philadelphia, Lippincott, 1998, p 505.

▷Mitchell C, Trampe B: Sonography and high-risk pregnancy. In Hagen-Ansert SL (ed): *Textbook of Diagnostic Ultrasonography*, 7th edition. St. Louis, Mosby Elsevier, 2012, p 1180.

210. D. Deuel's sign.

Deuel's sign, also known as the halo sign, is the halo effect that subcutaneous scalp edema produces on radiography of the fetal head. First described by Deuel on x-ray in 1946, Deuel's sign has been associated with intrauterine death of the fetus.

211. D. Chromosomal abnormalities.

Autosomal chromosomal abnormalities are rarely seen due to early fetal death therefore early pregnancy loss.

▷Bromley B, Benacerraf B: Chromosomal abnormalities. In Rumack CM, Wilson SR, Charboneau JW, et al (eds): *Diagnostic Ultrasound*, 4th edition. St. Louis, Elsevier Mosby, 2010, pp 1119–1144.

212. B. Abruption.

213. E. All of the above.

214. D. Retained products of conception (RPOC).

215. D. Pseudosac within endometrium with a + UCG.

216. C. Spaulding's sign.

217. D. M-mode.

218. B. Systole.

219. C. Diastole.

220. B. Failure of the cranial vault to form correctly.

    Holoprosencephaly is most commonly classified into one of three categorizes: alobar, semilobar, and lobar. The alobar and semilobar types are usually fatal. Although lobar holoprosencephaly is compatible with life, the child usually suffers from severe mental retardation.

▷Pilu G: Ultrasound evaluation of the fetal neural axis. In Callen PW (ed): *Ultrasonography in Obstetrics and Gynecology*, 5th edition. Philadelphia, Saunders Elsevier, 2008, pp 373–376.

221. B. Anencephaly.

222. A. Occipital region.

▷Saunders RC: *Clinical Sonography, A Practical Guide*, 3rd edition. Philadelphia, Lippincott, 1998, p 158.

▷Sanders RC: *Clinical Sonography: A Practical Guide*, 4th edition. Philadelphia, Lippincott, 2006.

223. B. Hydrocephalus.

224. C. Microcephaly.

Microcephaly is an abnormally small head (measuring 2 or more standard deviations below the mean), the result of an abnormally small brain. Severe microcephaly may be confused with anencephaly, but in microcephaly the cranial bones are present. In anencephaly there is absence of the cranial vault. Anencephaly—meaning absence of the brain—is associated and sometimes confused with acrania. Acrania—meaning without cranial bones— is the total or partial absence of the cranial bones. Because the fetal brain is exposed to amniotic fluid and deteriorates, acrania usually but not always develops into anencephaly.

▷Pilu G: Ultrasound evaluation of the fetal neural axis. In Callen PW (ed): *Ultrasonography in Obstetrics and Gynecology*, 5th edition. Philadelphia, Saunders Elsevier, 2008, pp 368–369, 382–385.

▷Henningsen CG: The fetal neural axis. In Hagen-Ansert SL (ed): *Textbook of Diagnostic Ultrasonography*, 7th edition. St. Louis, Mosby Elsevier, 2012, pp 1289–1310.

225. A. Encephalocele.

226. C. Arises from the cerebrum.

▷Pilu G: Ultrasound evaluation of the fetal neural axis. In Callen PW (ed): *Ultrasonography in Obstetrics and Gynecology*, 5th edition. Philadelphia, Saunders Elsevier, 2008, pp 377–380.

227. C. Dangling choroid.

The dangling choroid sign is a sonographic finding in ventriculomegaly (dilation of the ventricles within the fetal brain). The combination of ventriculomegaly and enlarged fetal head is hydrocephalus. The dangling choroid sign may be seen when the gravity-dependent choroid plexus falls into the enlarged space created by ventricular dilation.

▷Henningsen CG: The fetal neural axis. In Hagen-Ansert SL (ed): *Textbook of Diagnostic Ultrasonography*, 7th edition. St. Louis, Mosby Elsevier, 2012, pp 1289–1310.

228. C. Hydrocephalus.

229. A. Trisomy 13.

Holoprosencephaly is associated with chromosomal abnormalities, especially trisomy 13. There are other causes and associations as well, including a number of syndromes (Meckel's, Fryn's, Aicardi's, and hydrolethalus) and teratogens (alcohol, retinoic acid, phenytoin, maternal diabetes, and congenital infections). It is frequently associated with facial abnormalities. Other sonographic findings include IUGR, hydrocephaly, mircocephaly, and polyhydramnios. Defects of the fetal heart, kidneys, abdominal wall (omphalocele), neural tube (spina bifida) and gastrointestinal tract have also been found in the presence of holoprosencephaly.

One must always consider chromosomal abnormalities, trisomy 13 in particular, when there is holoprosencephaly. Holoprosencephaly results from abnormal cleavage of the fetal forebrain (the <u>prosencephalon</u>).

▷ Henningsen CG: The fetal neural axis. In Hagen-Ansert SL (ed): *Textbook of Diagnostic Ultrasonography*, 7th edition. St. Louis, Mosby Elsevier, 2012, pp 1289–1310.

230. E. A and C.

A fetus is considered macrosomic if it measures over the 90th percentile of weight for gestational age or if it weighs over 4000 grams at term.

▷Hickey J, Goldbey F: *Ultrasound Review of Obstetrics and Gynecology.* Philadelphia, Lippincott-Raven, 1996, p 161.

▷Benson CB, Doubilet PM: Fetal measurements: normal and abnormal fetal growth. In Rumack CM, Wilson SR, Charboneau JW, et al (eds): *Diagnostic Ultrasound*, 4th edition. St. Louis, Elsevier Mosby, 2010, p 1464.

231. C. Spina bifida.

Although it is nonspecific for spina bifida (failure of the neural tube to close), <u>the lemon sign</u>—a lemon-shaped head resulting from flattening of the frontal bone—is one of the cranial findings in spina bifida. Other sonographic cranial findings associated with spina bifida include dilated ventricles (ventriculomegaly), obliterated cisterna magna, and inferiorly displaced cerebellar vermis, giving the fetal cerebellum a rounded banana shape. Careful examination of the fetal spine in both transverse and sagittal views may demonstrate on or more findings that are specific for spinal bifida: (2) splayed posterior ossification centers in a V or U shape rather than the normal configuration of a circle, (2) open cleft in the skin overlying the fetal spine, and (3) protruding saclike structure over the spine.

▷Henningsen CG: The fetal neural axis. In Hagen-Ansert SL (ed): *Textbook of Diagnostic Ultrasonography*, 7th edition. St. Louis, Mosby Elsevier, 2012, pp 1289–1310.

232. B. Flattened cerebellum.

233. D. Choroid plexus cyst.

▷ Pilu G: Ultrasound evaluation of the fetal neural axis. In Callen PW (ed): *Ultrasonography in Obstetrics and Gynecology*, 5th edition. Philadelphia, Saunders Elsevier, 2008, pp 388–389.

234. D. Anencephaly.

235. D. A and B.

Fluid filling within the cranium can have differential diagnosis of either hydrocephalus or with hydranencephaly. The differences are that with massive hydrocephalus the ventricular atria fill with so much fluid that the normal brain anatomy is compromised and the fetal head is overall enlarged. The majority of the time cortical tissue can still be visualized. But in a case of hydranencephaly there is usually complete destruction of the fetal cortical brain tissue resulting in total atrophy of brain with replacement of this tissue with fluid.

▷Pilu G: Ultrasound evaluation of the fetal neural axis. In Callen PW (ed): *Ultrasonography in Obstetrics and Gynecology*, 5th edition. Philadelphia, Saunders Elsevier, 2008, pp 380–382.

236. B. Low-set ears.

Although it can be done it is very difficult to determine position of the fetal ears due to scanning error. Due to ultrasound being extremely angle and operator dependent the position of superficial structures in minimal degrees is very difficult.

▷Filly RA, Feldstein VA: Ultrasound evaluation of normal fetal anatomy. In Callen PW (ed): *Ultrasonography in Obstetrics and Gynecology*, 5th edition. Philadelphia, Saunders Elsevier, 2008, pp 300–302.

237. A. Encephalocele.

238. B. Absence of the nasal bridge.

This is a suboptimal image (the kind you may face on the exam).

239. D. Cyclopia.

240. C. Cyclopia.

241. B. Moderate posterior position of the mandible.

242. B. Turner's syndrome.

243. C. Cystic hygroma.

244. B. 15–21 weeks.

Not to be confused with nuchal translucency measurement, the nuchal fold, when thickened, is a soft marker for Down Syndrome in the second trimester and is measured at a different time than nuchal translucency, which is a method for identifying possible chromosomal abnormalities in the first trimester up to 14 weeks.

▷Chudleigh T, Thilaganathan B: *Obstetric Ultrasound: How, Why and When* 3rd edition. London, Elsevier Churchill Livingstone, 2004, p 118.

▷Malone FD: First trimester screening for aneuploidy. In Callen PW (ed): *Ultrasonography in* ▷*Obstetrics and Gynecology*, 5th edition. Philadelphia, Saunders Elsevier, 2008, pp 61–62.

245. C. Anencephaly.

246. B. Spina bifida.

247. D. Meningomyelocele.

248. B. Splaying of the laminae.

    In this image the three ossification centers of the fetal spine form a V rather than the circle that characterizes the normal sonographic presentation.

249. A. Cord insertion.

250. C. Omphalocele.

251. B. It is covered by peritoneum.

    Although other congenital anomalies are not usually associated with gastroschisis, bowel obstruction, premature deliveries, and low birth weights are. The exposed bowel can spill out protein into the amniotic fluid, and these pregnancies need to be monitored for growth restriction.

▷Bronshtein M, Blazer S, Zimmer EZ: The gastrointestinal tract and abdominal wall. In Callen PW (ed): *Ultrasonography in Obstetrics and Gynecology*, 5th edition. Philadelphia, Saunders Elsevier, 2008, pp 627–631.

252. E. Limb-body wall complex.

253. D. Fetal ascites.

254. D. A and B.

▷Bronshtein M, Blazer S, Zimmer EZ: The gastrointestinal tract and abdominal wall. In Callen PW (ed): *Ultrasonography in Obstetrics and Gynecology*, 5th edition. Philadelphia, Saunders Elsevier, 2008, pp 629–634.

255. C. Megacystis.

256. B. Can only be determined using biopsy.

▷Wladimiroff JW, Cohen-Overbeek TE, Laudy JAM: Ultrasound evaluation of the fetal thorax. In Callen PW (ed): *Ultrasonography in Obstetrics and Gynecology*, 5th edition. Philadelphia, Saunders Elsevier, 2008, pp 493, 501–502.

257. D. Diaphragmatic hernia.

258. C. Pleural effusion.

259. C. Pulmonary hyperplasia.

260. C. Hydronephrosis.

261. B. Polycystic kidney.

262. C. Posterior urethral valves obstruction (PUV).

Posterior urethral valves, which obstruct the posterior urethra, are the most common cause of bladder outlet obstruction in the male fetus. The sonographic presentation includes a persistent and oftentimes profoundly dilated bladder or thickened bladder walls. Distention of the posterior urethra is sometimes visualized, and moderate to severe oligohydramnios may be present when the obstruction affects the fetus's ability to void into the amniotic sac, as is often the case. Although obstruction of the bladder outlet mainly affects the male fetus, the female fetus also may suffer from urethral obstruction secondary to a number of pathologies. In the female, the most common cause of urethral obstruction is cloacal malformation or urethral atresia.

▷Avni FE, Maugey-Laulom B, Cassart M, et al: The fetal genitourinary tract. In Callen PW (ed): *Ultrasonography in Obstetrics and Gynecology*, 5th edition. Philadelphia, Saunders Elsevier, 2008, p 649.

▷Fong KW, Robertson J, Maxwell CV: The fetal urogenital tract. In Rumack CM, Wilson SR, Charboneau JW, et al (eds): *Diagnostic Ultrasound*, 4th edition. St. Louis, Elsevier Mosby, 2010, pp 1353–1388.

263. D. Ureteropelvic junction obstruction.

264. D. Unilateral ureteropelvic junction (UPJ) obstruction.

Unilateral ureteropelvic junction obstruction, the most common cause of hydronephrosis in the neonate, is caused by a congenital obstruction of urine flow from the renal pelvis into the ureter; it is characterized by dilation of the pelvis and the calyces. Because the contralateral kidney is normal, amniotic fluid remains normal. Oligohydramnios is unusual. So is bilateral UPJ obstruction, but in rare cases of severe bilateral UPJ obstruction oligohydramnios can develop as a late feature.

▷Avni FE, Maugey-Laulom B, Cassart M, et al: The fetal genitourinary tract. In Callen PW (ed): *Ultrasonography in Obstetrics and Gynecology*, 5th edition. Philadelphia, Saunders Elsevier, 2008, pp 767–770.

265. A. Classic Potter's syndrome.

266. B. Urachal cyst.

Early in the development of the embryo the allantois develops from the hindgut. It is continuous with the bladder and projects into the connecting stalk. The blood vessels of the allantois become those of the umbilical cord. The allantois regresses to become the urachus, a fibrous cord or ligament extending from the apex of the bladder to the umbilicus. Rarely, instead of regressing and developing into a ligament, the allantoid lumen may persist as a patent canal connection from the bladder to the umbilicus, into which urine then drains. If a smaller part of the original allantois remains, it becomes an urachal cyst. In the adult, the urachus persists as the median umbilical ligament. It runs just under the abdominal wall from the superior bladder dome to the umbilicus.

▷Rosenberg HK, Chaudhry H: Pediatric pelvic sonography. In Rumack CM. Wilson SR, Charboneau JW, et al (eds): *Diagnostic Ultrasound*, 4th edition. St. Louis, Elsevier Mosby, 2010, pp 1925–1981.

▷Callen PW (ed): *Ultrasonography in Obstetrics and Gynecology*, 5th edition Philadelphia. Saunders Elsevier, 2008, pp 664–665, 745.

▷Hagen-Ansert SL: The fetal urogenitary system. In Hagen-Ansert SL (ed): *Textbook of Diagnostic Ultrasonography*, 7th edition. St. Louis, Mosby Elsevier, 2012, pp 1350–1379.

267. B. Hydronephrosis.

268. E. All of the above.

The fetal heart should occupy one-third of the fetal chest and be positioned at a 45° angle to the left of fetal midline. This position will show the right ventricle to be closest to the anterior chest wall and the left atrium closest to the aorta. Non-visualization of the fetal stomach in association with excess amniotic fluid should prompt the consideration of esophageal atresia.

▷Stamm ER, Drose JA: The fetal heart. In Rumack CM, Wilson SR, Charboneau JW, et al (eds): *Diagnostic Ultrasound*, 4th edition. St. Louis, Elsevier Mosby, 2010, pp 1294–1326.

269. D. A and B.

270. D. Down's syndrome.

Other findings associated with Down's syndrome include slightly shortened femur, mild pelviectasis, thickened nuchal fold, brachycephaly, duodenal atresia, and congenital heart defects.

▷Benacherraf B: *Ultrasound of Fetal Syndromes.*
New York, Churchill Livingston, 1998, p 416.

▷Benacherraf B: *Ultrasound of Fetal Syndromes,*
2nd edition. New York, Churchill Livingston, 2007.

271. B. Dilated duodenum next to the fetal stomach.

272. D. Artifact or dysplasia.

Bowing of the femur on the sonogram may represent dysplasia or artifact. Side lobe or grating lobe are off-axis artifacts. That is, they emanate from the transducer at an angle to the main beam rather than in line with the main beam. Side lobes occur with all transducers, while grating lobes are produced only by array transducers. Both side and grating lobes are weaker than the main lobe (or beam), but when they are intense enough they produce noise and artifacts in the image, including lateral displacement of particularly strong reflections (echoes) received by the transducer. When energy from these side or grating lobes strikes a strongly reflective interface such as bone, the transducer may receive and display the echo in the image. But since the off-axis side and grating lobes course at an angle to the main beam, the actual location of the interface is not displayed. The ultrasound system must always assume that echoes are reflected from the main lobe of energy, and so it displays off-axis lobe reflections with a lateral displacement. These artifacts can cause the fetal femur to appear bowed or even fractured. Changing the angle of insonation and making other probe adjustments can correct the artifactual bowing.

▷Kremkau FW: *Sonography: Principles and Instruments*, 8th edition. Philadelphia, Saunders Elsevier, 2011, pp 176–210.

273. C. Osteogenesis imperfecta and artifact.

▷Gonçalves L, Kusanovic JP, Gotsch F, et al: The fetal musculoskeletal system. In Callen PW (ed): *Ultrasonography in Obstetrics and Gynecology*, 5th edition. Philadelphia, Saunders Elsevier, 2008. pp 453–454.

274. B. Clubfoot.

275. E. All of the above.

▷Gill K: Diabetes mellitus and pregnancy. Ob-Gyn Ultrasound Today, Lesson 10, Volume 3, 1998.

276. C. Cloverleaf.

Strawberry head shape is seen in a fetus with Trisomy 18 (Edward's syndrome). Multiple fetal anomalies are usually associated with Trisomy 18—most of them involving the face, brain, heart, and extremities—and this abnormally shaped head

is almost always seen with marked abnormalities. The strawberry shape of the head can appear very similar to the lemon sign seen in patients with open neural tube defects. The difference is that the cerebellum in these strawberry-shaped heads is normal.

The lemon-shaped fetal skull (sonographically, the <u>lemon sign</u>) is very commonly imaged in the fetus with open neural tube defects. It is the shape a sonographer will most often encounter together with the banana sign. The <u>banana sign</u> is the shape that the cerebellum assumes as the neural structures are pulled out of their normal position.

When the head is longer than usual in the transverse plane (BPD) and shorter than usual in the anteroposterior plane (OFD), the "short" head shape is termed <u>brachycephaly</u>. Brachycephaly is not always abnormal. In fact, certain races (native American, Malayan, and Burmese among them) are typically and normally brachycephalic. It is the cephalic index that is used to determine normality, as well as to avoid overestimation of gestational age in brachycephaly. In dolichocephaly, where the head shape is longer than usual (i.e., shorter in the transverse plane and longer in the anteroposterior plane), gestational age may be underestimated. Again, the cephalic index is used to determine normality of fetal head shape:

$$CI = BPD \div OFD$$

Normal CI is 80%, and range of normal is 75% to 85%. A cephalic index of less than 75% suggests dolichocephaly, while one exceeding 85% suggests brachycephaly. See also answers 122 and 123 above.

<u>Frontal bossing</u> is an abnormal protrusion and rounding of the frontal bones of a fetus that is usually seen in <u>achondroplasia</u>, the most common skeletal dysplasia.

▷Benacerraf B: *Ultrasound of Fetal Syndromes*. New York, Churchill Livingston, 1998, pp 12–13, 332.

▷Benacherraf B: *Ultrasound of Fetal Syndromes*, 2nd edition. New York, Churchill Livingston, 2007.

▷Glanc P, Chitayat D, Unger S: The fetal musculoskeletal system. In Rumack CM, Wilson SR, Charboneau JW, et al (eds): *Diagnostic Ultrasound*, 4th edition. St. Louis, Elsevier Mosby, 2010, pp 1389–1423.

▷DuBose TJ, Hagen-Ansert SL: Obstetric measurements and gestational age. In Hagen-Ansert SL (ed): *Textbook of Diagnostic Ultrasonography*, 7th edition. St. Louis, Mosby Elsevier, 2012, pp 1142–1157.

277. D. Overlapping digits.

278. E. B and C.

▷Benacherraf B: *Ultrasound of Fetal Syndromes.* New York, Churchill Livingston, 1998, pp 250–253, 384.

▷Benacherraf B: *Ultrasound of Fetal Syndromes*, 2nd edition. New York, Churchill Livingston, 2007.

279. E. Sandal gap deformity.

Hand and foot abnormalities are frequently associated with chromosomal abnormalities particularly when associated with other abnormal findings.

▷Saunders RC: *Clinical Sonography: A Practical Guide*, 3rd edition. Philadelphia, Lippincott, 1998, pp 136–137.

▷Sanders RC: *Clinical Sonography: A Practical Guide*, 4th edition. Philadelphia, Lippincott, 2006.

280. C. Rocker bottom.

▷Saunders RC: *Clinical Sonography: A Practical Guide*, 3rd edition. Philadelphia, Lippincott, 1998, pp 136–137.

▷Sanders RC: *Clinical Sonography: A Practical Guide*, 4th edition. Philadelphia, Lippincott, 2006.

281. C. Hypoplastic left ventricle.

▷Stamm ER, Drose JA: The fetal heart. In Rumack CM, Wilson SR, Charboneau JW, et al (eds): *Diagnostic Ultrasound*, 4th edition. St. Louis, Elsevier Mosby, 2010, pp 1294–1326.

282. B. Congenital diaphragmatic hernia.

In the normal fetus a primitive diaphragm has formed by the 8th menstrual week. Normal formation involves a complex process in which four structures fuse: (1) the septum transversum, (2) pleuroperitoneal membranes, (3) dorsal mesentery of the esophagus, and (4) body ball. It is thought that the failure of these four structures to fuse completely leads to the herniation of abdominal organs and structures into the thorax. Congenital diaphragmatic hernias (CDHs), the most common developmental abnormality of the diaphragm, may be central in location at the foramen of Morgagni or located at the lateral corners at the foramen of Bochdalek, which is the most common. Most are left-sided (75—90%). Right-sided CDHs occur in approximately 10% of cases. Bilateral CDHs are rare, with an incidence of less than 5%, and difficult to detect sonographically because there is no or little cardiomediastinal shift.

▷Wladimiroff JW, Cohen-Overbeek TE, Laudy JAM: Ultrasound evaluation of the fetal thorax. In Callen PW (ed): *Ultrasonography in Obstetrics and* ▷*Gynecology*, 5th edition. Philadelphia, Saunders Elsevier, 2008, pp 505–507.

283. C. Transposition of the great vessels.

▷ Stamm ER, Drose JA: The fetal heart. In Rumack
CM, Wilson SR, Charboneau JW, et al (eds):
Diagnostic Ultrasound, 4th edition. St. Louis, Elsevier
Mosby, 2010, pp 1294–1326.

284. D. Pericardial effusion.

285. A. Are common and benign.

Isolated premature contractions of the fetal heart are common, transitory, almost always benign, and rarely require treatment. Complications after birth are rare as well. There are three main kinds of isolated premature contractions: (1) premature atrial contractions, which account for the great majority of fetal rhythm irregularities; (2) premature ventricular contractions, which are less common; and (3) premature junctional contractions, in which there is simultaneous atrial and ventricular contraction. Normally, the electrical events that produce the mechanical contractions proceed first from atrial sinus activity, then to atrioventricular nodal activity, and lastly to ventricular activity.

The heart rate of the normal fetus varies from 110 to 180 beats per minute. Fetal heart rates that are abnormally fast or slow indicate other kinds of rhythm disturbances. The tachyarrhythmias (supraventricular tachycardia is the most common presentation) are characterized by an abnormally fast rhythm of > 200 bpm. Bradyarrhythmia is characterized by an abnormally slow rhythm of < 100 bpm.

▷ Yoo SJ, Jaeggi E: Ultrasound evaluation of the
fetal heart. In Callen PW (ed): *Ultrasonography in
Obstetrics and Gynecology*, 5th edition. Philadelphia,
Saunders Elsevier, 2008, pp 572–573.

286. B. Down's syndrome.

▷Benacherraf B: *Ultrasound of Fetal Syndromes*.
New York, Churchill Livingston, 1998, pp 328–336,
404.

▷Benacherraf B: *Ultrasound of Fetal Syndromes*,
2nd edition. New York, Churchill Livingston, 2007.

287. C. Trisomy 21.

▷Benacherraf B: *Ultrasound of Fetal Syndromes*.
New York, Churchill Livingston, 1998, pp 328–336,
404.

▷Benacherraf B: *Ultrasound of Fetal Syndromes*,
2nd edition. New York, Churchill Livingston, 2007.

288. B. Proboscis.

289. C. Beckwith-Wiedemann syndrome.

Beckwith-Wiedemann syndrome was first described in the 1960s as a syndrome associated with gigantism, macroglossia, omphaloceles, and renal abnormalities.

▷Benacherraf B: *Ultrasound of Fetal Syndromes.*
New York, Churchill Livingston, 1998, pp 93–95.

▷Benacherraf B: *Ultrasound of Fetal Syndromes,*
2nd edition. New York, Churchill Livingston, 2007.

290. B. Classic Potter's syndrome.

Classic Potter's syndrome refers to bilateral renal agenesis. Besides the fact that we cannot live without our kidneys, the severe oligohydramnios associated with the process inhibits normal development of the fetal lungs.

▷Benacherraf B: *Ultrasound of Fetal Syndromes.*
New York, Churchill Livingston, 1998, pp 272–274.

▷Benacherraf B: *Ultrasound of Fetal Syndromes,*
2nd edition. New York, Churchill Livingston, 2007.

291. D. Cystic hygroma.

▷Benacherraf B: *Ultrasound of Fetal Syndromes.*
New York, Churchill Livingston, 1998, pp 340–342.

▷Benacherraf B: *Ultrasound of Fetal Syndromes,*
2nd edition. New York, Churchill Livingston, 2007.

292. C. Trisomy 21.

The thickened nuchal fold was first described and associated with Down's syndrome (trisomy 21) in 1985. It is considered to be the single most sensitive and specific sonographic marker for detecting this syndrome during the second trimester. Nuchal folds greater than or equal to 6 mm have detected 40–70% of affected fetuses with a false-positive rate of less than 1%. This finding tends to resolve and become less reliable later in pregnancy.

▷Benacherraf B: *Ultrasound of Fetal Syndromes.*
New York, Churchill Livingston, 1998, p 335.

▷Benacherraf B: *Ultrasound of Fetal Syndromes,*
2nd edition. New York, Churchill Livingston, 2007.

293. D. Triploidy.

The <u>normal human karyotype</u> has 46 chromosomes, 22 pairs of autosomes, and one pair of sex chromosomes. In the aneuploid conditions—trisomy 13, trisomy 18, trisomy 21 (Down's syndrome), and Turner's syndrome are the big ones—there is too much or too little chromosomal material. Trisomy 21, for instance, is characterized by an extra chromosome 21. In <u>triploidy</u>, there is an entire extra set of chromosomes, often the result of two sperm fertilizing the ovum. **<u>Exam tip:</u>** *Note the key word "set" in the question.*

▷Henningsen CG: Prenatal diagnosis of congenital anomalies. In Hagen-Ansert SL (ed): *Textbook of Diagnostic Ultrasonography,* 7th edition. St. Louis, Mosby Elsevier, 2012, pp 1190–1205.

294. B. Cystic hygroma, webbed neck, and infantile sexual characteristics.

▷Benacerraf BR: Sonographic diagnosis of syndromes of the fetus. In Fleischer AC, Manning FA, Jeanty P, et al: *Sonography in Obstetrics and Gynecology: Principles & Practice*, 5th edition. Stamford, CT, Appleton & Lange, 1996, p 503.

▷Henningsen CG: Prenatal diagnosis of congenital anomalies. In Hagen-Ansert SL (ed): *Textbook of Diagnostic Ultrasonography*, 7th edition. St. Louis, Mosby Elsevier, 2012, p 1204.

295. D. Flat nasal profile, duodenal atresia, ventriculomegaly, and echogenic bowel.

296. B. Potter's syndrome.

297. F. Spalding's sign.

298. B. Skin edema.

299. D. Trophoblastic disease.

AFP is produced by the fetal liver and excreted into the amniotic fluid. Through diffusion across the placenta, it gets into the maternal bloodstream. In certain conditions, abnormal amounts of AFP are spilled out and increase the MSAFP.

▷ Norton ME: Genetics and prenatal diagnosis. In Callen PW (ed): *Ultrasonography in Obstetrics and Gynecology*, 5th edition. Philadelphia, Saunders Elsevier, 2008, pp 42–46.

300. D. Gestational diabetic.

301. C. S/D ratio.

The systolic/diastolic ratios are important most often in the high-risk population for proving intrauterine growth restriction (IUGR). A waveform is most commonly taken from the umbilical artery, and these waveforms show marked decrease in the systolic flow in patients with IUGR.

▷Galan HL, Pandipati S, Filly RA: Ultrasound evaluation of fetal biometry and normal and abnormal fetal growth. In Callen PW (ed): *Ultrasonography in Obstetrics and Gynecology*, 5th edition. Philadelphia, Saunders Elsevier, 2008, pp 247–250.

302. C. Fetal hydrops.

When the sonographer visualizes two or more sites at which fluid has collected in the fetus, fetal hydrops (or hydrops fetalis) is considered to exist. These abnormal collections of fluid may include pleural effusions, pericardial effusions, abdominal ascites, hydroceles, and anasarca (skin edema).

303. B. IUP with hemorrhagic cyst.

304. C. Hydatidiform mole.

305. A. Uterine fibroid.

306. E. 16 weeks.

Corpus luteum cysts, like the corpus luteum of pregnancy, tend to regress as the end of the first trimester nears. Follow-up evaluation at the beginning of the second trimester (14 menstrual weeks) usually shows the lesion to be regressing or gone.

▷Filly RA: Ultrasound evaluation during the first trimester. In Callen PW (ed): *Ultrasonography in Obstetrics and Gynecology*, 3rd edition. Philadelphia, WB Saunders, 1994, pp 82–83.

▷Goldstein C, Hagen-Ansert SL, Vander Werff BJ: Pathology of the ovaries. In Hagen-Ansert SL (ed): *Textbook of Diagnostic Ultrasonography*, 7th edition. St. Louis, Mosby Elsevier, 2012, p 1007.

307. C. Fetal demise.

308. C. 16–20 weeks.

Laparotomy for ovarian masses is usually not conducted until the mid second trimester (after the 18th week), provided, of course, that the operation can be postponed until then.

▷Filly RA: Ultrasound evaluation during the first trimester. In Callen PW (ed): *Ultrasonography in Obstetrics and Gynecology*, 3rd edition. Philadelphia, WB Saunders, 1994, pp 82–83.

309. A. Leiomyoma.

Leiomyomas are the most common solid mass encountered during pregnancy. Increased hormone levels during pregnancy enlarge pre-existing fibroids.

▷Hickey J, Goldberg F: *Ultrasound Review of Obstetrics and Gynecology*. Philadelphia, Lippincott-Raven, 1996, p 38.

▷Poder L: Ultrasound evaluation of the uterus. In Callen PW (ed): *Ultrasonography in Obstetrics and Gynecology*, 5th edition. Philadelphia, Saunders Elsevier, 2008, p 930.

310. B. Corpus luteum cyst.

311. E. Theca lutein cysts.

Theca lutein cysts are caused by abnormally high levels of hCG associated with gestational trophoblastic disease, ovarian hyperstimulation, multiple pregnancy, and choriocarcinoma.

▷Hickey J, Goldberg F: *Ultrasound Review of Obstetrics and Gynecology*. Philadelphia, Lippincott-Raven, 1996, p 44.

▷Sebire NJ: Gestational trophoblastic neoplasia. In Callen PW (ed): *Ultrasonography in Obstetrics and*

Gynecology, 5th edition. Philadelphia, Saunders
Elsevier, 2008, pp 951–967.

312. C. Focal myometrial contractions.

Focal myometrial contractions are painless, localized contractions of the myometrium that occur throughout pregnancy and are not always clinically apparent. Not to be confused with Braxton-Hicks contractions, where the entire uterus contracts similar to that during delivery.

▷Hickey J, Goldberg F: *Ultrasound Review of Obstetrics and Gynecology.* Philadelphia, Lippincott-Raven, 1996, p 37.

GYNECOLOGY

313. A. Foley catheter.

314. B. Solid.

315. C. Pouch of Douglas.

316. D. Adrenal.

317. E. Piriformis.

318. B. Piriformis.

319. D. In the ampulla.

320. A. Mid-cycle.

321. E. Premenstrual syndrome.

Although the corpus luteum cyst produces some estrogen, the main hormone produced is progesterone. Progesterone is responsible for the symptoms of pregnancy, such as nausea, fatigue, and breast tenderness. It also is responsible for the irritability, breast tenderness, and water retention associated with PMS.

322. C. Levator ani muscles.

323. E. 5 mm.

Postmenopausal women should have a double-layer thickness less than 5 mm. Patients on tamoxifen therapy and women taking hormone supplements postmenopausally are allowed a normal thickness up to 8 mm.

▷Johnson PT, Kurtz AB: *Case Review: Obstetrical and Gynecologic Ultrasound.* St. Louis, Mosby, 2001, p 56.

▷Reuter K, Babagbemi TK: *Obstetric and Gynecologic Ultrasound: Case Review Series.* St. Louis, Mosby, 2006.

324. B. Internal iliac artery.

The internal iliac artery, vein, and ureter can be seen coursing posterior to the ovary; however, the artery is immediately posterior to the ovary, followed by the vein and ureter.

325. C. High-velocity, high-resistance pattern.

326. D. Low-velocity, low-resistance pattern.

▷Levi CS, Lyons EA, Holt SC, et al: Normal anatomy of the female pelvis and transvaginal sonography. In Callen PW (ed): *Ultrasonography in Obstetrics and Gynecology,* 5th edition. Philadelphia, Saunders Elsevier, 2008, pp 898–905.

327. A. Urinary tract.

The gonads and urinary tract develop at the same time in the pelvic compartment. For this reason, anomalies of one system often affect the other.

328. E. 3600.

329. B. 1800.

330. C. Hyperstimulated.

Normal follicles should show ovarian parenchyma between them. If no ovarian tissue can be seen between the cysts and the cysts are relatively equal in size, one should suspect hyperstimulation.

331. A. Vagina.

332. B. Obturator internus.

333. B. Anteflexed.

Filling the urinary bladder provides easier sonographic access by flattening the uterus so that the sound beam is perpendicular to the uterine surfaces.

334. D. Vagina.

335. E. Parietalis.

336. C. They are benign, common, and frequently multiple.

The nabothian cyst is an obstructed and dilated endocervical gland. These cysts are common findings in the reproductive age group and are best visualized with

endovaginal scans that demonstrate one or more small simple cysts within the wall of the cervix. Nabothian cysts are mostly clinically insignificant.

▷Sauerbrei EE: The nongravid uterus, vagina, and urethra. In Sauerbrei EE, Nguyen KT, Nolan RL: *A Practical Guide to Ultrasound in Obstetrics and Gynecology*, 2nd Edition. Philadelphia, Lippincott-Raven, 1998, p 51.

▷Goldstein C, Hagen-Ansert SL: Pathology of the uterus. In Hagen-Ansert SL (ed): *Textbook of Diagnostic Ultrasonography*, 7th edition. St. Louis, Mosby Elsevier, 2012, p 979.

337. C. Lateral.

338. D. Fallopian tubes are routinely imaged sonographically.

Normal fallopian tubes are not routinely seen with ultrasound, transabdominally or transvaginally, because they are very narrow in diameter and surrounded by bowel. If they become swollen or dilated they will appear as tubular structures in the adnexal regions, often in the cul-de-sac region.

339. C. Dilated veins.

Engorged pelvic vasculature is not an uncommon finding, especially in the reproductive years. Engorged and varicose veins may cause pelvic pressure or pain, a condition commonly referred to as pelvic congestion.

340. A. Smaller.

Although the uterus involutes after pregnancy, it never shrinks back to the original size. If the muscular organ has been stretched several times it will lose some elasticity. A general rule is that you can add approximately 0.5–1 cm per pregnancy to each measurement (longitudinal, transverse, AP). *This should be taken into consideration when evaluating the uterus of a multigravid patient.*

341. C. Nonvisualized.

342. D. Posterior, anterior.

343. D. The ureter and iliac vessels are posterior to the ovary.

344. E. Bowel.

345. B. 8 x 3 x 4 cm.

346. E. Mullerian.

347. D. Patient with a large fibroid uterus.

348. C. Can penetrate up to 12 cm depth.

Transvaginal transducers range from 5–7.5 MHz. These high-frequency transducers provide excellent resolution but poor penetration, allowing visualization of only a couple of inches deep. Large masses cannot be adequately evaluated with this technique.

349. A. Betadine.

350. B. Globular.

The term globular means globe-like or rounded.

351. C. Anterior reverberation artifact.

When the transducer is close to a fluid-filled structure, the common reverberation artifact occurs, particularly when the ultrasound beam is perpendicular to the structure. A strong echo is produced at the highly reflective interface. As it returns to the transducer it can be redirected back into the patient, where it is reflected again. The back-and-forth reverberation creates the soft specular reflections in the anterior portion of the fluid collection.

352. C. Left ovary.

353. B. Hyperstimulated.

354. A. Internal iliac artery.

355. D. Retroflexed.

356. A. Isthmus.

The isthmus of the uterus is sometimes referred to as the neck or lower uterine segment. It is the junction between the cervix and corpus where you see the uterus bend.

357. D. It is a major suspensory ligament for the uterus.

The broad ligament is actually a double fold of peritoneum and does not provide a solid means of suspension for the uterus.

358. D. Internal iliac.

359. A. Cervical.

360. E. Fornix.

361. A. Fill the bladder.

362. A. Proliferative.

363. C. Leiomyoma.

364. B. Anterior myometrium.

365. C. Periovulatory.

366. D. Anteflexed.

367. E. Ililpsoas muscles.

368. C. Isthmus.

369. B. Graafian follicle.

A preantral follicle is a developing follicle. If fertilization does not occur, the corpus luteum becomes the corpus albicans as it regresses. Upon fertilization, the corpus luteum persists to produce progesterone that helps to maintain the pregnancy until the placenta can take over the function. Theca lutein cysts are bilateral and correspond to hyperstimulated ovaries.

370. D. 2.5 cm.

Once the dominant follicle is recognized, its size may be followed to the immediate preovulatory period. During this time the follicle grows rapidly in a linear manner, by 2–3 mm a day, and reaches a mean diameter of about 20–24 mm by the time of ovulation.

▷Levi CS, Lyons EA, Holt SC, et al: Normal anatomy of the female pelvis. In Callen PW (ed): *Ultrasonography in Obstetrics and Gynecology*, 5th edition. Philadelphia, Saunders Elsevier, 2008, pp 910–911.

371. B. Periovulatory.

372. D. 24–36 hours.

373. C. Dermoid cyst.

374. E. Estrogen.

It is estrogen that acts on the female reproductive system to create the environment necessary for fertilization, implantation, and nutrition of the early embryo. During the follicular phase of the menstrual cycle (days 1–14, which includes both the menstrual phase [days 1–4] and the proliferative phase [days 5 to 15]), the pituitary gland produces follicle-stimulating hormone (FSH). As its name indicates, FSH stimulates the rapid growth of a mature follicle in the ovary. The growing follicle elaborates estrogen, which by approximately day 5 stimulates the proliferation and thickening of the functional layer of endometrium in preparation for implantation of a fertilized ovum. The endometrial lining continues to thicken throughout days 15–28 of the menstrual cycle (the secretory or luteal phase).

Without fertilization and pregnancy, the endometrial lining thins markedly during days 1–4 of the new menstrual phase.

▷Tempkin BB, Bizjak PM: The female pelvis. In Curry RA, Tempkin BB (eds): *Sonography: Introduction to Normal Structure and Function*, 3rd edition. Philadelphia, Elsevier Saunders, 2011, p 358.

375. D. 4000.

376. A. Human choriogonadotropin (hCG).

Following implantation of the fertilized ovum, human choriogonadotropin (hCG) is secreted by the developing placenta.

▷Tempkin BB, Bizjak PM: The female pelvis. In Curry RA, Tempkin BB (eds): *Sonography: Introduction to Normal Structure and Function*, 3rd edition. Philadelphia, Elsevier Saunders, 2011, pp 376–377.

377. B. Corpus luteal cyst.

The pill (oral contraceptive) prevents ovulation. FSH (follicle stimulating hormone) secretion is depressed and the LH peak is abolished.

▷Govan ADT, Hodge C, Callander R: *Gynecology Illustrated*, 3rd edition. New York, Churchill-Livingstone, 1985, p 406.

▷Bain C, Burton K, McGavigan J: *Gynaecology Illustrated*, 6th edition. New York, Churchill-Livingstone, 2011.

▷Bain C, Burton K, McGavigan J, et al: *Gynaecology Illustrated*, 6tj edition. New York, Churchill-Livingstone, 2011, pp 343–345.

378. D. Menarche.

379. D. During the periovulatory stage.

380. B. 2–3 mm.

381. E. Secretory phase.

382. A. 1–2 weeks.

383. C. Combination oral contraceptives.

384. B. Zygote.

385. D. Pituitary.

Follicle Stimulating Hormone (FSH) is a gonadotropin produced by the anterior pituitary gland that initiates follicular development.

▷Tempkin BB, Bizjak PM: The female pelvis. In Curry RA, Tempkin BB (eds): *Sonography: Introduction to Normal Structure and Function*, 3rd edition. Philadelphia, Elsevier Saunders, 2011, p 376.

386. C. 48.

387. C. ½.

388. A. Increase to a point and then plateau.

389. C. 8 mm.

390. C. Clean smooth walls.

391. C. 28.

Between puberty and menopause, the female reproductive system normally undergoes monthly cyclical changes. The menstrual cycle usually follows a 28-day course, during which a single ovum reaches maturity and is released into the genital tract.

▷Tempkin BB, Bizjak PM: The female pelvis. In Curry RA, Tempkin BB (eds): *Sonography: Introduction to Normal Structure and Function*, 3rd edition. Philadelphia, Elsevier Saunders, 2011, p 376.

392. A. LH.

FSH—follicle stimulating hormone—is produced by the pituitary gland and stimulates follicular development and the secretion of estrogen. LH—luteinizing hormone—is a gonadotropin that stimulates ovulation and the secretion of estrogen and progesterone. It too is produced by the pituitary gland. PAPPA—pregnancy-associated plasma protein—is a biochemical measurement used to assess risks for chromosomal defects.

393. D. Progesterone.

394. E. Proliferative.

395. C. Mittleschmertz.

Mid-cycle pain (mittleschmertz) is associated with pelvic inflammation but may occur alone. It is sometimes accompanied by slight vaginal staining and is caused by changes in estrogen levels. The word is German and is translated as middle pain.

▷Miller BF, Keane CB: *Encyclopedia and Dictionary of Medicine, Nursing and Allied Health*, 7th edition. Philadelphia, WB Saunders, 2003, p 1135.

▷Govan ADT, Hodge C, Callander R: *Gynecology Illustrated*, 3rd edition. New York, Churchill-Livingstone, 1985, p 121.

▷Bain C, Burton K, McGavigan J: *Gynaecology Illustrated*, 6th edition. New York, Churchill-Livingstone, 2011.

396. D. Placenta.

397. B. 14.

398. E. Cystadenoma.

399. C. Ovary and adrenal gland.

400. A. Amenorrhea.

401. A. Menopause.

402. D. Secretory.

403. B. Retroflexed.

404. B. Corpus luteum cyst.

405. D. Engorged vessels.

406. E. Pituitary gland.

FSH and LH are produced by the anterior pituitary gland in response to the influence of Gn-RH produced by the hypothalamus. FSH causes the ovarian follicles to enlarge and LH induces ovulation of the dominant follicle.

407. D. 14 days.

The life of the corpus luteum is approximately 14 days after ovulation. If fertilization does not occur, it will begin to regress into the corpus albicans. Upon fertilization, the ovum begins producing hCG which inhibits the corpus luteum from regressing and it continues to produce estrogen and progesterone until the trophoblastic cells of the placenta are able to produce enough hormones to sustain the pregnancy.

408. E. Hematocolpos.

The most common cause for hematocolpos in a patient of this age would be the imperforate hymen. Other causes include gynetresia or traumatic stenosis from radiation scarring.

409. D. Adrenal hyperplasia.

410. B. Hematometracolpos.

411. C. Imperforate hymen.

412. A. Pelvic inflammatory disease.

413. D. Granulosa cell tumor.

Granulosa theca cell tumor is the most common stromal tumor in children. It is often associated with feminizing effects and precocious puberty as a result of estrogen production.

▷Rosenberg HK, Chaudhry H: Pediatric pelvic
sonography. In Rumack CM, Wilson SR,
Charboneau JW, et al (eds): *Diagnostic Ultrasound*,
4th edition. St. Louis, Elsevier Mosby, 2010, pp
1925–1981.

414. E. Turner's syndrome.

415. C. The cervix occupies most of the length of the uterine body until puberty.

INFANTILE (6 weeks–2 years): The cervix is longer comprising 2/3 total length of the uterine body, and there is no flexion between the cervix and the uterus. CHILDHOOD (2 years–menarche): Tubular or inverse pear-shaped uterus that persists in this appearance until puberty.

▷Callen PW (ed): *Ultrasonography in Obstetrics and
Gynecology*, 5th edition. Philadelphia, Saunders
Elsevier, 2008, p 1049.

▷Hickey J, Goldberg F: *Ultrasound Review of
Obstetrics and Gynecology*. Philadelphia, Lippincott-
Raven, 1996, p 20.

416. A. Mixed gonadal dysgenesis.

▷ DeLange M, Rouse GA: *Ob/Gyn Sonography: An
Illustrated Review*. Pasadena, CA, Davies
Publishing, 2004, p 241.

417. C. Intrauterine device.

418. E. All of the above.

▷DeLange M, Rouse GA: *Ob/Gyn Sonography: An
Illustrated Review*. Pasadena, CA, Davies
Publishing, 2004, p 245.

419. B. Anovulation.

420. D. Hysterosalpingography.

421. D. Hydrosalpinx.

422. C. Endometriosis.

▷Westphalen AC, Qayyum A: The role of magnetic resonance imaging in the evaluation of gynecologic disease. In Callen PW (ed): *Ultrasonography in Obstetrics and Gynecology*, 5th edition. Philadelphia, Saunders Elsevier, 2008, p 1060.

423. D. After sexual intercourse.

424. C. Estrogen.

425. A. Preovulatory.

426. B. Endometrial polyp.

427. E. Clomid.

Clomid, the brand name for clomiphene citrate, is useful in stimulating ovulation in patients who fail to ovulate because of hypothalamic or pituitary problems. Administered orally early in the menstrual cycle, it suppresses circulating estrogen, "tricking" the pituitary gland into releasing additional follicular stimulating hormone and luteinizing hormone. The FSH and LH stimulate the ovary to ripen a follicle and release an egg.

▷Pierson RA: Ultrasonographic imaging in infertility. In Callen PW (ed): *Ultrasonography in Obstetrics and Gynecology*, 5th edition. Philadelphia, Saunders Elsevier, 2008, p 999.

428. A. hCG.

Human chorionic gonadotropin (hCG; brand names Profasi, Pregnyl) acts to mature the developing follicle and trigger the release of an egg. It is administered by intramuscular injection.

429. E. Limited field of view.

430. D. Hyperstimulation.

431. B. Estradiol.

▷Riddle AF, Sharma V: In vitro fertilization and other assisted conception techniques. In Chervenask FA, Isaacson G, Campbell S (eds): *Ultrasound in Obstetrics and Gynecology*, Volume 2. Boston, Little, Brown, 1993, pp 1705–1710.

432. A. Permits the physician to retrieve many oocytes.

▷Fleischer AC, Vasquez J: Transvaginal sonography scanning in gynecologic infertility. In Fleischer AC, Manning FA, Jeanty P, et al (eds): *Sonography in Obstetrics and Gynecology Principles & Practice*, 5th edition. Samford, CT, Appleton & Lange, 1996, pp 914–916.

▷Mitchell C, Trampe B, Lebovic D: The role of ultrasound in evaluating female infertility. In Hagen-Ansert S (ed): *Textbook of Diagnostic Ultrasonography*, 7th edition. St. Louis, Mosby Elsevier, 2012, pp 1044–1045.

433. E. A and C.

▷De Lange M, Rouse GA: Infertility. In: *Ob/Gyn Sonography: An Illustrated Review*. Pasadena, CA, Davies Publishing, 2004, p 252.

▷Riddle AF, Sharma V: In vitro fertilization and other assisted conception techniques. In Chervenask FA, Isaacson G, Campbell S (eds): *Ultrasound in Obstetrics and Gynecology*, Volume 2. Boston, Little, Brown, 1993, pp 1705–1710.

434. C. ZIFT.

▷De Lange M, Rouse GA: Infertility. In: *Ob/Gyn Sonography: An Illustrated Review*. Pasadena, CA, Davies Publishing, 2004, p 252.

▷Riddle AF, Sharma V: In vitro fertilization and other assisted conception techniques. In Chervenask FA, Isaacson G, Campbell S (eds): *Ultrasound in Obstetrics and Gynecology*, Volume 2. Boston, Little, Brown, 1993, pp 1705–1710.

435. A. Endometrial fluid collections are common.

Postmenopausal endometrial fluid is usually due to atrophy and degeneration of the endometrium resulting in a serous type fluid contained in the cavity.

▷Vander Werff BJ, Hagen-Ansert: Pathology of the uterus. In Hagen-Ansert S (ed): *Textbook of Diagnostic Ultrasonography*, 7th edition. St. Louis, Mosby Elsevier, 2012, pp 978–1000.

436. D. Thin.

437. E. 8 mm.

438. C. 5 mm.

439. D. They can always be identified transvaginally.

▷Middleton WD, Kurtz AB, Hertzberg BS: *Ultrasound: The Requisites*, 2nd edition. St. Louis, Mosby, 2004, p 563.

440. C. Endometrial carcinoma.

441. A. Benign hyperplasia.

Although endometrial hyperplasia is pathologically benign, it is considered a precursor to endometrial cancer and is usually treated similarly.

442. D. Endometriosis.

Endometriosis and its symptoms rely on hormone stimulation. In the absence of hormone production, as seen in postmenopausal women, the process and symptoms subside.

443. B. Endometrial.

Adenocarcinoma of the endometrium is the most common gynecologic cancer in the United States today. Over the past 50 years the incidence of endometrial carcinoma has been rising, while the incidence of cervical carcinoma has been declining.

▷Westphalen AC, Qayyum A: The role of MRI in the evaluation of gynecologic disease. In Callen PW (ed): *Ultrasonography in Obstetrics and Gynecology*, 5th edition. Philadelphia, Saunders Elsevier, 2008, p 1065.

444. A. It decreases in size and is infantile in appearance.

445. C. Low impedance.

▷Fleischer A, Kepple DM: Color Doppler sonography of pelvic masses. In Fleischer AC, Manning FA, Jeanty P, et al (eds): *Sonography in OB/GYN: Principles and Practice*, 6th edition. New York, McGraw-Hill, 2001, pp 802–808.

446. D. Endometrial atrophy.

447. B. Ovarian fibroma.

Hydrothorax may accompany ascites due to any cause, or may occur as an accompaniment of a lung tumor. The so-called Meigs' syndrome describes the specific condition of ascites and hydrothorax in conjunction with a benign ovarian fibroma.

▷Borok KK: Ovarian mass. In Henningsen C: *Clinical Guide to Ultrasonography.* St. Louis, Mosby, 2004, pp 228, 240.

▷Govan ADT, Hodge C, Callander R: *Gynecology Illustrated*, 3rd edition. New York, Churchill-Livingstone, 1985, p 346.

▷Bain C, Burton K, McGavigan J: *Gynaecology Illustrated*, 6th edition. New York, Churchill-Livingstone, 2011.

448. A. Ovary.

449. D. Cystadenoma.

450. D. Dysgerminoma.

451. B. Cystic and ovarian in origin.

452. B. Endometrioma.

453. C. Large, thick-walled cyst with multiple thick septations and free fluid.

    Benign masses are usually cystic and the walls of the mass are thin. If septations are present, they are thin and lack solid tissue growth or papillary projections. Size may be relevant with most benign masses measuring less than 5 cm.

    ▷Westphalen AC, Qayyum A: The role of MRI in the evaluation of gynecologic disease. In Callen PW (ed): *Ultrasonography in Obstetrics and Gynecology*, 5th edition. Philadelphia, Saunders Elsevier, 2008, pp 1067–1073.

454. D. Endoderm, mesoderm, and ectoderm.

455. A. Ectoderm.

    Although the terms dermoid and cystic teratoma are often interchanged, they are pathologically different. The ectoderm is the outermost of the three primitive germ layers of the embryo; from it are derived the epidermis and epidermic tissues such as hair, nails, glands of the skin, the nervous system, external sensory organs, and mucous membranes of the mouth and anus.

    ▷ Miller BF, Keane CB, O'Toole MT: *Encyclopedia & Dictionary of Medicine, Nursing & Allied Health*, 7th Edition. St. Louis, Saunders Elsevier, 2005, p 493.

456. C. Obesity, hirsutism, and infertility.

    Stein-Leventhal syndrome is associated with polycystic ovary disease. Due to anovulation from hormone imbalances, the patient often gives a history of infertility. Menses may not occur regularly, and some patients may menstruate only once or twice a year. Excessive androgen production causes hirsutism. Obesity is common, but not always present.

    ▷Kunau-Szczesniak PA: Infertility. In Henningsen C: *Clinical Guide to Ultrasonography*. St. Louis, Mosby, 2004, pp 217–219.

    ▷Govan ADT: *Gynecology Illustrated*, 3rd edition. New York, Churchill-Livingstone, 1985, pp 109–111.

    ▷Bain C, Burton K, McGavigan J: *Gynaecology Illustrated*, 6th edition. New York, Churchill-Livingstone, 2011.

457. E. Benign and estrogenic.

    Granulosa cell tumors may be discovered in patients of all ages, including children, but mostly are seen in postmenopausal patients. They are usually benign but do have malignant potential. These estrogenic tumors secrete estrogen, causing secondary female characteristics that present as precocious puberty in children and cause vaginal bleeding and breast dysplasia in the postmenopausal patient.

458. E. Leiomyoma.

459. B. Arrhenoblastoma.

Arrhenoblastomas are androgenic tumors that secrete testosterone, causing secondary male characteristics. Female patients present with a masculine stature and male hair growth patterns on the face, abdomen, and upper thighs. After removal, female characteristics should return.

460. A. Lymph nodes.

Tumor first directly invades neighboring structures—peritoneum, uterus, bladder, bowel and omentum. Second is transcoelomic metastasis along paracolonic gutters. Third, the tumor invades the lymphatic system. Finally, malignant cells are borne by blood to liver and lungs, usually late in the disease process.

▷Govan ADT: *Gynecology Illustrated*, 3rd edition. New York, Churchill-Livingstone, 1985, p 361.

▷Bain C, Burton K, McGavigan J: *Gynaecology Illustrated*, 6th edition. New York, Churchill-Livingstone, 2011.

461. A. Mullerian ducts.

462. D. Space of Retzius.

463. A. Paraovarian cyst.

Paraovarian cysts, sometimes referred to as broad ligament cysts, arise from the epoophoron. The epoophoron lies in the mesosalpinx and then parallel to the uterus. Other cysts found in the mesosalpinx and around the terminal portion of the fallopian tube are called cysts of Kobelt's tubules, hydatids of Morgagni, or fimbrial cysts.

▷Borok KK: Ovarian mass. In Henningsen C: *Clinical Guide to Ultrasonography.* St. Louis, Mosby, 2004, p 232.

▷Govan ADT: *Gynecology Illustrated*, 3rd edition. New York, Churchill-Livingstone, 1985, pp 320–321.

▷Bain C, Burton K, McGavigan J: *Gynaecology Illustrated*, 6th edition. New York, Churchill-Livingstone, 2011.

464. E. Associated with multiparity.

Patients with endometriosis often complain of infertility. This condition seems to be more prevalent among upper middle class professional women who have delayed childbearing until careers are established. This delay contributes to the difficulty of becoming pregnant.

465. E. Menorrhagia, dysmenorrhea, dyspareunia, and cyclic pain.

466. A. Anterior and superior.

467. B. It is a metastatic tumor from a GI tract primary.

468. A. It is a malignant tumor of the endometrium.

469. C. Leiomyoma.

   A benign tumor made of connective and muscle tissue, the leiomyoma is considered the most common uterine tumor with 20–40% incidence in the female population.

470. E. All of the above.

471. B. Uterine fibroids.

472. A. Fibroid uterus.

473. C. Vagina.

474. E. Bicornuate uterus.

475. B. Ovaries.

476. B. Polycystic ovaries.

477. A. Hydrosalpinx.

478. D. Exposure to DES (diethylstilbesterol).

479. A. Nausea and vomiting.

480. C. Multiple gestations.

   Women whose mothers used DES during pregnancy can have a T-shaped uterus or uterine cavity constrictions that are not amenable to surgical correction. In addition, they have an increased risk of cervical and vaginal malignancies.

   ▷Johnson PT, Kurtz AB: *Case Review: Obstetric and Gynecologic Ultrasound.* St. Louis, Mosby, 2001, p 28.

   ▷Reuter K, Babagbemi TK: *Obstetric and Gynecologic Ultrasound: Case Review Series.* St. Louis, Mosby, 2006.

481. A. Inhibit spontaneous abortion.

   DES was used in the 1940s and 1950s in high-risk pregnancies—diabetes, habitual abortion, threatened abortion and other obstetrical risk situations—to prevent pregnancy wastage.

▷Miller BF, Keane CB, O'Toole MT: *Encyclopedia & Dictionary of Medicine, Nursing & Allied Health*, 7th Edition. St. Louis, Saunders Elsevier, 2005, p 514.

▷Beck WW: *Obstetrics and Gynecology-The National Medical Series for Independent Study*. New York, John Wiley & Sons, 1986, pp 308–309.

▷Pfeifer SM: *NMS Obstetrics and Gynecology (National Medical Series for Independent Study)*, 7th edition. Philadelphia, Lippincott Williams & Wilkins, 2011.

482. C. Cervix.

483. C. Most are benign.

484. B. Ovarian fibroma.

The so-called Meigs' syndrome describes the specific condition of ascites and hydrothorax in conjunction with a benign ovarian fibroma.

▷Borok KK: Ovarian mass. In Henningsen C: *Clinical Guide to Ultrasonography*. St. Louis, Mosby, 2004, p 228.

▷Govan ADT, Hodge C, Callander R: *Gynecology Illustrated*, 3rd edition. New York, Churchill-Livingstone, 1985, p 346.

▷Bain C, Burton K, McGavigan J: *Gynaecology Illustrated*, 6th edition. New York, Churchill-Livingstone, 2011.

485. A. Pelvic inflammatory disease.

PID or salpingo-oophoritis is generally preceded by vaginal and cervical colonization of pathogenic bacteria, a state that may exist for months or years. Development of perihepatitis with adhesions and right upper quadrant abdominal pain is known as the Fitz-Hugh Curtis syndrome.

▷Swearengin R: Pelvic inflammatory disease. In Henningsen C: *Clinical Guide to Ultrasonography*. St. Louis, Mosby, 2004, pp 206–211.

▷Beck WW: *Obstetrics and Gynecology: The National Medical Series for Independent Study*. Media, PA, Harwal Publishing, 1986, p 216.

▷Pfeifer SM: *NMS Obstetrics and Gynecology (National Medical Series for Independent Study)*, 7th edition. Philadelphia, Lippincott Williams & Wilkins, 2011.

486. D. Right upper quadrant pain and PID.

▷Swearengin R: Pelvic inflammatory disease. In Henningsen C: *Clinical Guide to Ultrasonography*. St. Louis, Mosby, 2004, pp 206–211.

▷Beck WW: *Obstetrics and Gynecology: The National Medical Series for Independent Study.* Media, PA, Harwal Publishing, 1986, p 216.

▷Pfeifer SM: *NMS Obstetrics and Gynecology (National Medical Series for Independent Study)*, 7th edition. Philadelphia, Lippincott Williams & Wilkins, 2011.

487. E. Urinary obstruction, kidneys.

488. E. All of the above.

489. C. Hydronephrosis.

490. B. Always check Morison's pouch.

Morison's pouch is the hepatorenal space.

491. D. Malignancy.

492. E. Pelvic ascites.

493. D. Metastatic liver disease.

494. B. Fitz-Hugh Curtis syndrome.

Near the level of the fallopian tubes there is a communication between the abdominal and pelvic compartments. This is why fluids such as ascites and blood can migrate into the upper abdominal quadrants. If untreated, pelvic inflammation can migrate and cause inflammation around the liver and could ultimately lead to peritonitis.

495. D. Meigs' syndrome.

496. D. Pelvic ascites.

497. A. Slice thickness artifact.

It is important to recognize this artifact because it can interject misleading echoes where there should be none, making a cyst appear to contain echoes or a bladder appear to contain debris. Simply changing the transducer position or angle will eliminate the artifact.

498. B. Hepatic adenoma.

PATIENT CARE, PREPARATION, TECHNIQUE

499. C. C.

500. D. D.

501. B. B.

502. A. A.

503. C. In the left upper corner of the image.

504. D. Retroflexed.

> ▷Fleischer AC, Toy EC, Wesley L, et al (eds):
> *Sonography in Obstetrics and Gynecology, Principles
> and Practice*, 7th edition. Columbus, OH, McGraw-
> Hill Professional, 2011.

505. A. Supine hypotensive syndrome.

506. E. Roll her on her left side.

507. D. Magnifies the pelvic organs.

508. A. Lithotomy.

509. D. Cephalic presentation, longitudinal lie, spine on maternal right.

*Fetal lie and presenting anatomy can be determined on the basis of the sonographic
plane and the fetal anatomy (spine, stomach on left, gallbladder on right). By
convention, the image is viewed and interpreted as though from the mother's feet
upward. Therefore, you know that the fetus is in a longitudinal lie, cephalic
presentation, with its spine on the maternal right:*

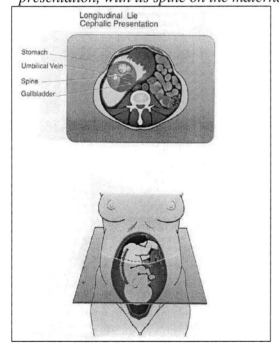

510. B. Breech presentation, longitudinal lie, spine on maternal left.

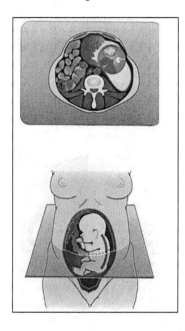

511. C. Frank breech.

Frank breech (in which the fetal thighs are flexed at the hips with legs and knees extended, as illustrated here) is most common. It is also the least likely to involve cord prolapse; the greatest risk of cord prolapse is with footling breach. Complete breech is the least common of the breech presentations.

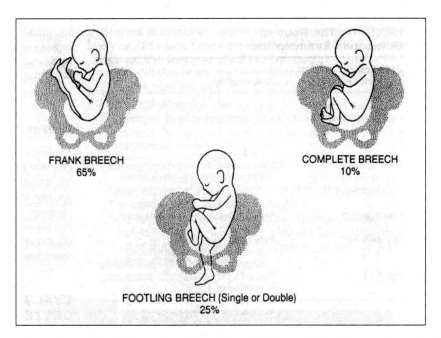

FRANK BREECH
65%

COMPLETE BREECH
10%

FOOTLING BREECH (Single or Double)
25%

Illustration reprinted with permission from Callen PW: The obstetrical ultrasound examination. In Callen PW (ed): *Ultrasonography in Obstetrics and Gynecology*, 4th edition. Philadelphia, WB Saunders, 2000, p 13.

▷Hickey J, Goldberg F: *Ultrasound Review of Obstetrics and Gynecology*. Philadelphia, Lippincott-Raven, 1996, p 159.

▷ Callen PW: The obstetric ultrasound examination. In Callen PW (ed): *Ultrasonography in Obstetrics and Gynecology*, 5th edition. Philadelphia, Saunders Elsevier, 2008, pp 14–16.

512. B. Transverse lie with head on maternal left.

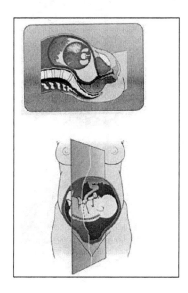

Illustration reprinted with permission from Callen PW: The obstetrical ultrasound examination. In Callen PW (ed): *Ultrasonography in Obstetrics and Gynecology*, 4th edition. Philadelphia, WB Saunders, 2000, p 12.

513. A. Transverse lie with head on maternal right.

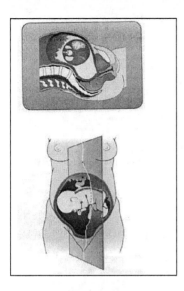

Illustration reprinted with permission from Callen PW: The obstetrical ultrasound examination. In Callen PW (ed): *Ultrasonography in Obstetrics and Gynecology*, 4th edition. Philadelphia, WB Saunders, 2000, p 12.

514. E. There is an ectopic pregnancy identified in the right adnexa.

Some institutions require sonographers to write a technical impression after the examination is completed. This impression should describe the location, size, and echogenicity of any abnormal findings. The sonographer should not write a diagnosis or differential diagnosis.

▷Tempkin BB, Gill KA: First scanning experience. In Curry RA, Tempkin BB: *Sonography: Introduction to Normal Structure and Function*, 3rd edition. Philadelphia, Elsevier Saunders, 2011, p 56.

PART V

Application for CME Credit

Objectives of this Activity
How To Obtain CME Credit
Applicant Information
Evaluation—You Grade Us!
CME Quiz

This continuing medical educational (CME) activity is approved for 12 hours of credit by the Society of Diagnostic Medical Sonography. This credit may be applied as follows:

- Sonographers and technologists may apply these hours toward the CME requirements of the ARDMS, ARRT, and/or CCI, as well as to the CME requirements of ICAVL for technologists and sonographers in ICAVL-accredited facilities.

- Physicians may apply a certain maximum number of SDMS-approved credit hours toward the CME requirements of the ICAVL for accreditation of diagnostic facilities. (Be sure to confirm current requirements with the pertinent organizations.) Physicians who are registered sonographers or technologists may apply all of these hours toward the CME requirements of the ARDMS, ARRT, and/or CCI. SDMS-approved credit is not applicable toward the AMA Physician's Recognition Award.

If you have any questions about CME requirements that affect you, please contact the responsible organization directly for current information. CME requirements can and sometimes do change.

OBJECTIVES OF THE ACTIVITY

Upon completion of this educational activity, you will be able to:

1 Describe and identify normal and abnormal fetal and female pelvic anatomy and physiology.
2 Describe how, when, and why ultrasonography is applied in the practice of obstetrics and gynecology.
3 Differentiate normal from abnormal obstetrical and gynecologic sonographic findings and explain the correlations between these findings and pertinent laboratory and imaging studies.
4 Describe how, when, and why fetal and gynecological measurements are made.
5 Explain the role of medical genetics in the practice of obstetrics and gynecology.
6 Describe the diseases, disorders, complications, and coexisting disorders of the female reproductive system, pregnancy, and antepartum and postpartum fetus.

7   Explain how to prepare for, perform, and explain the techniques of sonographic examination in the practice of obstetrics and gynecology.

HOW TO OBTAIN CME CREDIT

1   Read and study the book and complete the interactive exercises it contains.
2   Photocopy and then complete the applicant information page, evaluation questionnaire (you grade us!), and answer sheet.
3   Make copies of the completed forms for your records and then return the originals (i.e., the photocopied forms with your original writing) to the following address for processing:

> **Davies Publishing, Inc.**
> **Attn: CME Coordinator**
> **32 South Raymond Avenue, Suite 4**
> **Pasadena, California 91105-1935**
>
> **Or fax to (626)792-5308**

You may also fax us the applicable pages and pay by credit card. Our fax number is 626-792-5308. Call us with your credit card, expiration date, and 3- or 4-digit security code or include it with the fax. We grade quizzes within 24 hours of receipt and will email and mail your certificate. Questions? Please call us at 626-792-3046.

4   If more than one person will be applying for credit, be sure to photocopy the applicant information, evaluation form, and CME quiz so that you always have the original on hand for use.

APPLICANT INFORMATION

Name _____ Date of birth _____

Current credentials _____

Home address _____

City/State/Zip _____

Telephone _____ eMail address _____

ARDMS # _____ ARRT # _____ CCI# _____ SDMS# _____

Check _____ Credit Card _____ Exp Date _____

3- or 4-digit security code _____ Signature certifying your completion of the activity _____

NOTE

The original purchaser of this CME activity is entitled to submit this CME application for an administrative fee of $39.50. Please enclose a check payable to Davies Publishing Inc. with your application. Others may also submit applications for CME credits by completing the activity as explained above and enclosing an administrative fee of $49.50. The CME administrative fee helps to defray the cost of processing, evaluating, and maintaining a record of your application and the credit you earn. Fees may change without notice. For the current fee, call us at 626.792.3046, e-mail us at **cme@DaviesPublishing.com**, or write to us at the aforementioned address. We will be happy to help!

ANSWER SHEET

///

Circle the correct answer below and return this sheet to Davies Publishing Inc. Passing criterion is 70%. Applicant may have no more than 3 attempts to pass.

1. A B C D E	41. A B C D E	81. A B C D E
2. A B C D E	42. A B C D E	82. A B C D E
3. A B C D E	43. A B C D E	83. A B C D E
4. A B C D E	44. A B C D E	84. A B C D E
5. A B C D E	45. A B C D E	85. A B C D E
6. A B C D E	46. A B C D E	86. A B C D E
7. A B C D E	47. A B C D E	87. A B C D E
8. A B C D E	48. A B C D E	88. A B C D E
9. A B C D E	49. A B C D E	89. A B C D E
10. A B C D E	50. A B C D E	90. A B C D E
11. A B C D E	51. A B C D E	91. A B C D E
12. A B C D E	52. A B C D E	92. A B C D E
13. A B C D E	53. A B C D E	93. A B C D E
14. A B C D E	54. A B C D E	94. A B C D E
15. A B C D E	55. A B C D E	95. A B C D E
16. A B C D E	56. A B C D E	96. A B C D E
17. A B C D E	57. A B C D E	97. A B C D E
18. A B C D E	58. A B C D E	98. A B C D E
19. A B C D E	59. A B C D E	99. A B C D E
20. A B C D E	60. A B C D E	100. A B C D E
21. A B C D E	61. A B C D	101. A B C D E
22. A B C D E	62. A B C D E	102. A B C D E
23. A B C D E	63. A B C D E	103. A B C D E
24. A B C D E	64. A B C D E	104. A B C D E
25. A B C D E	65. A B C D E	105. A B C D E
26. A B C D E	66. A B C D E	106. A B C D E
27. A B C D E	67. A B C D E	107. A B C D E
28. A B C D E	68. A B C D E	108. A B C D E
29. A B C D E	69. A B C D E	109. A B C D E
30. A B C D E	70. A B C D E	110. A B C D E
31. A B C D E	71. A B C D E	111. A B C D E
32. A B C D E	72. A B C D E	112. A B C D E
33. A B C D E	73. A B C D E	113. A B C D E
34. A B C D E	74. A B C D E	114. A B C D E
35. A B C D E	75. A B C D E	115. A B C D E
36. A B C D E	76. A B C D E	116. A B C D E
37. A B C D E	77. A B C D E	117. A B C D E
38. A B C D E	78. A B C D E	118. A B C D E
39. A B C D E	79. A B C D E	119. A B C D E
40. A B C D E	80. A B C D E	120. A B C D E

Evaluation—You Grade Us!

/ /

Please let us know what you think of *Ob/Gyn Sonography Review*. **Participating in this quality survey is a requirement for CME applicants, and it benefits future readers by ensuring that current readers are satisfied and, if not, that their comments and opinions are heard and taken into account. Your opinions count!**

1 Why did you purchase *Ob/Gyn Sonography Review*? (Circle primary reason.)

   REGISTRY REVIEW   COURSE TEXT   CLINICAL REFERENCE   CME ACTIVITY

2 Have you used *Ob/Gyn Sonography Review* for other reasons, too? (Circle all that apply.)

   REGISTRY REVIEW   COURSE ACTIVITY   CLINICAL REFERENCE   CME ACTIVITY

3 To what extent did *Ob/Gyn Sonography Review* meet its stated objectives and your needs? (Circle one.)

   GREATLY   MODERATELY   MINIMALLY   INSIGNIFICANTLY

4 The content of *Ob/Gyn Sonography Review* was (circle one):

   JUST RIGHT   TOO BASIC   TOO ADVANCED

5 The quality of the questions and explanations was mainly (circle one):

   EXCELLENT   GOOD   FAIR   POOR

6 The manner in which *Ob/Gyn Sonography Review* presents the material is mainly (circle one):

   EXCELLENT ·   GOOD   FAIR   POOR

7 If you used this book to prepare for the registry exam, did you also use other materials or take any exam-preparation courses?

   NO   YES (PLEASE SPECIFY WHAT MATERIALS AND COURSES)

   _____

   _____

8 If you used this book for a course, please name the course, the instructor's name, the name of the school or program, and any other textbooks you may have used:

   COURSE/INSTRUCTOR/SCHOOL OR PROGRAM:

   _____

   _____

   OTHER TEXTBOOKS:

   _____

   _____

9   What did you like best about *Ob/Gyn Sonography Review*?

_____
_____
_____

10 What did you like least about *Ob/Gyn Sonography Review*?

_____
_____
_____

11 If you used *Ob/Gyn Sonography Review* to prepare for the ARDMS exam in
    OB/GYN, did you pass?

    YES   NO   HAVEN'T YET TAKEN IT

12 May we quote any of your comments in our catalogs or promotional material?

    YES   NO   FURTHER COMMENT . . .

_____
_____
_____
_____
_____
_____
_____
_____
_____
_____
_____
_____
_____
_____

CME QUIZ

Please answer the following questions after you have completed the CME activity. There is one <u>best</u> answer for each question. Circle it on the answer sheet that appears on the previous page.

1.   A yolk sac is considered abnormal when its diameter exceeds:

    A. 2 mm
    B. 3 mm
    C. 4 mm
    D. 5 mm
    E. 6 mm

2.   The term *double bleb sign* refers to the:

    A. The amnion and yolk sac
    B. Two intrauterine gestational sacs
    C. The amnion and chorion
    D. A heterotopic pregnancy
    E. A bicornuate uterus

3.   The segment of the fallopian tube that is potentially the most life-threatening in a ruptured ectopic pregnancy is:

    A. Interstitial
    B. Ampulla
    C. Isthmus
    D. Fimbria
    E. Ligamentous

4.   Because of spinal segmentation, crown-rump length measurements begin to lose accuracy after:

    A. 3 weeks
    B. 5 weeks
    C. 7 weeks
    D. 9 weeks
    E. 11 weeks

5.   Why is nuchal translucency measured?

    A. It is a good indicator of gestational age.
    B. It is a good indicator of possible chromosomal abnormalities.
    C. It is a good indicator of possible placenta abruption.
    D. It is an indicator of possible neural tube defects.
    E. It is of no practical significance.

6.   Normally, nuchal translucency does not exceed:

    A. 1 mm
    B. 2 mm

C. 3 mm

D. 4 mm

E. 6 mm

7. Normal measurements for the lateral ventricle of the fetal brain are:

A. 1 cm in the largest dimension longitudinally

B. 1 cm in the largest dimension transversely

C. 10 mm in the largest dimension longitudinally

D. 1 mm in the largest dimension transversely

E. B and D

8. Normally, the anatomic structure closest to the spine in a four-chamber view of the fetal heart is the:

A. Right atrium

B. Left ventricle

C. Right ventricle

D. Left atrium

E. Apex

9. In the fetal heart, the communication between the right and left atria is termed:

A. Ventricular septal defect

B. Atrial septal defect

C. Atrial orifice

D. Foramen ovale

E. Atrial meatus

10. You visualize a small, rounded echogenic structure within the left ventricle of a fetal heart. You suspect:

A. Aortic semilunar valve

B. Ventricular septum

C. CHF

D. Left ventricular embolus

E. Chordae tendineae

11. In which plane is the diaphragm best visualized?

A. Longitudinal

B. Oblique to the fetus' left

C. Transverse

D. Oblique to the fetus' right

E. Coronal

12. The fluid-filled stomach should always be visualized in the fetal left upper quadrant. If it is not seen during the course of an exam, one should suspect:

A. Pyloric stenosis

B. Duodenal atresia

    C. Jejunoileal obstruction
    D. Esophageal atresia
    E. Ulcerative colitis

13. The bladder of the male fetus is sometimes enlarged because of:

    A. Imperforate hymen
    B. Glans imperfecta
    C. Posterior urethral valves
    D. Ureteropelvic junction
    E. Megacystis

14. Second trimester obstetrical ultrasound examinations are best in determining:

    A. Gestational age of the fetus
    B. Fetal birth weight
    C. Fetal position
    D. Fetal anatomy
    E. Fetal life

15. Characteristics of a biophysical profile include:

    A. Fetal breathing
    B. Fetal tone
    C. Fetal movement
    D. Amniotic fluid index
    E. All of the above

16. A placenta previa can be ruled out if the placental edge is at least this distance from the internal cervical os.

    A. 0.5 cm
    B. 1 cm
    C. 1.5 cm
    D. 2 cm
    E. 3 cm

17. You are unable to identify the vascular space between placenta and myometrium. You suspect:

    A. Placenta accreta
    B. Abruption placenta
    C. Marginal placenta previa
    D. Succenturiate placenta
    E. Vasa previa

18. A patient presents with severe abdominal pain and vaginal bleeding. This sonogram demonstrates:

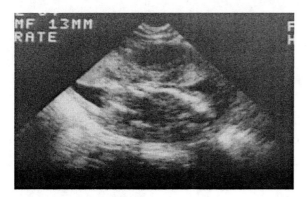

A. Placenta previa
B. Circumvallate placenta
C. Placental abruption
D. Marginal placenta
E. Normal placenta

19. The best method and time for estimating gestational age would be:

    A. Gestational sac measurement at 5 weeks
    B. Crown-rump length at 10 weeks
    C. Biparietal diameter at 15 weeks
    D. Abdominal circumference at 20 weeks
    E. Femur length at 30 weeks

20. The best way to determine fetal lung maturity is:

    A. Biometric evaluation
    B. Echogenicity of lungs
    C. Chorionic villus sampling
    D. Alphafetoprotein levels
    E. Amniocentesis

21. With normal growth during the first trimester, the size of the gestational sac should increase daily by:

    A. 1 mm
    B. 2 mm
    C. 5 mm
    D. 10 mm
    E. 1 cm

22. The long bone LEAST likely to be affected by intrauterine growth restriction the:

    A. Femur
    B. Humerus
    C. Tibia
    D. Clavicle
    E. Radius

23. Twins resulting from the fertilization of a single ova are referred to as:

    A. Monozygotic
    B. Dizygotic
    C. Monoamniotic
    D. Dichorionic
    E. Fraternal

24. If a patient's AFP level is low, one should check for:

    A. Neural tube defects
    B. Multiple gestation
    C. Abdominal wall defects
    D. Trisomy 21
    E. Skeletal dysplasia

25. This image leads you to suspect:

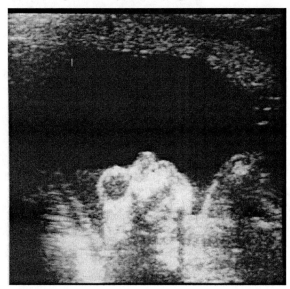

    A. Hydrocephalus
    B. Acrania
    C. Anencephaly
    D. Encephalocele
    E. Cleft palate

26. The following transverse image is from a patient who presents large for gestational age at 7–8 weeks LMP. The image demonstrates:

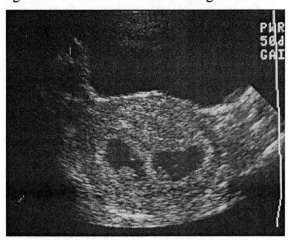

    A. Polyhydramnios
    B. Single sac with implantation bleed
    C. Split image artifact
    D. Bicornuate uterus
    E. Twins

27. The term puerperium refers to which period?

    A. Before delivery
    B. First trimester
    C. Second trimester
    D. Third trimester
    E. After delivery

28. A McDonald's procedure is performed to:

    A. Remove an IUD
    B. Freeze the cervix for dysplasia
    C. Treat an incompetent cervix
    D. Treatment to enhance fertility
    E. Artificially inseminate

29. The quantitative method of determining whether the amniotic fluid level is normal or not is called:

    A. Amniotic fluid index
    B. Eyeballing
    C. Qualitative evaluation
    D. Amniocentesis
    E. Uterine volume

30. Amniotic fluid is produced by the:

    A. Fetal liver
    B. Fetal kidneys
    C. Fetal gut
    D. Placenta
    E. Choroids plexus

31. What does a triple marker screening (triple test) measure?

    A. Unconjugated estriol (uE3)
    B. Acetylcholinesterase (ACHE)
    C. Human chorionic gonadotropin (hCG)
    D. Alpha-fetoprotein (AFP)
    E. A, C, and D

32. For which of the following is acetycholinesterase (ACHE) most specific?

    A. Down's syndrome
    B. Spina bifida
    C. Trisomy 13
    D. Trisomy 18
    E. Triploidy

33. During the first trimester the most common cause of fetal demise is:

    A. Maternal uterine anomalies
    B. Chromosomal abnormalities
    C. Maternal diabetes mellitus
    D. Intrauterine infections
    E. Unknown cause

34. Which of the following is the result of a defect in the cranium and herniation of cranial meninges through the defect?

    A. Encephalocele
    B. Daryocystoceles
    C. Cystic hygroma
    D. Holoprosencephaly
    E. Anencephaly

35. Holoprosencephaly is most often associated with which of the following?

    A. Triploidy
    B. Trisomy 13
    C. Trisomy 18
    D. Trisomy 21
    E. Down's syndrome

36. Which of the following statements about hydranencephaly is TRUE?

    A. Poor prognosis
    B. Complete destruction of the cerebrum
    C. Bilateral clefts in the cerebrum
    D. A and B
    E. A and C

37. What is NOT associated with fetal hydrops?

    A. Pleural effusion
    B. Megacystis
    C. Anasarca
    D. Ascites
    E. Pericardial effusion

38. In an unborn fetus, the most common renal abnormality is:

    A. Multicystic kidney
    B. Polycystic kidney
    C. Hydronephrosis
    D. Potter's syndrome Type I
    E. Potter's syndrome Type II

39. Which of the following conditions can be ruled out by visualizing the fetal heart and stomach in their correct positions?

    A. Congenital diaphragmatic hernia
    B. Duodenal atresia
    C. Situs inversus
    D. A and B
    E. All of the above

40. What is meant by the term *double bubble*?

    A. Fetal stomach next to heart
    B. Dilated duodenum next to the fetal stomach
    C. Bilateral hydronephrosis
    D. Choledochal cyst next to stomach
    E. Urachal cyst next to bladder

41. Double right outlet is almost always associated with:

    A. Pulmonary atresia
    B. Aortic stenosis
    C. Hypoplastic left ventricle
    D. Arrhythmia
    E. Premature ventricular contractions (PVC)

42. Brightly echogenic bowel may be associated with:

    A. Down's syndrome
    B. Turner's syndrome
    C. Classic Potter's syndrome
    D. Fetal alcohol syndrome
    E. Duodenal atresia

43. Anasarca is:

    A. Scalp edema
    B. Skin edema
    C. Overlapping of cranial bones
    D. Overlapping of the digits
    E. Fetal decay

44. In which of the following conditions is MSAFP NOT elevated?

    A. Multiple gestation
    B. Anencephaly
    C. Omphalocele
    D. Trophoblastic disease
    E. Spina bifida

45. Your patient presents at 14 weeks LMP large for gestational age and bleeding. Heart tones cannot be heard. You suspect:

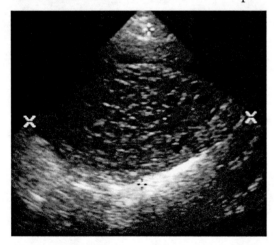

    A. Fetal demise
    B. Premature rupture of membranes
    C. Placental abruption
    D. Placenta previa
    E. Hydatidiform mole

46. In a pregnant woman with a pelvic mass that requires surgical intervention, the best time to operate would be:

    A. 6–8 weeks
    B. 10–12 weeks
    C. 16–20 weeks
    D. 24–32 weeks
    E. At term

47. What is the term for the uterine contractions commonly seen during obstetrical sonography?

    A. Braxton-Hicks contractions
    B. Diffuse endometrial contractions
    C. Focal myometrial contractions
    D. Fitshugh-Curtis contractions
    E. Labor contractions

48. Which muscles are most frequently mistaken for enlarged ovaries?

    A. Obturator internus
    B. Piriformis
    C. Iliopsoas
    D. Levator ani
    E. Coccygeus

49. Estrogen is NOT responsible for:

    A. Premenstrual syndrome
    B. Inducing rhythmic contraction of the fallopian tubes
    C. Causing fibroids to enlarge
    D. Breast duct engorgement
    E. Stimulating endometrial proliferation

50. What forms the floor of the pelvis?

    A. Piriformis muscles
    B. Iliopsoas muscles
    C. Levator ani muscles
    D. Obtlurator internus muscles
    E. Coccygeus muscles

51. Ovarian arterial flow is typically:

    A. Low-velocity, high-resistance pattern
    B. High-velocity, low-resistance pattern
    C. High-velocity, high-resistance pattern
    D. Low-velocity, low-resistance pattern
    E. Reverse-flow pattern

52. All of these statements about the fallopian tubes are true EXCEPT:

    A. They lie within the broad ligament.
    B. Fertilization usually occurs within the ampullary portion.
    C. The tube provides nutrients for the ova and sperm.
    D. Fallopian tubes are routinely imaged sonographically.
    E. The fimbria communicates with the peritoneal cavity.

53. Sonographically, how will the uterus of a nulliparous female appear compared to that of a multiparous female?

    A. Smaller
    B. Larger
    C. More dense
    D. Flatter
    E. More globular

54. Which part of the uterus is the least distinctive part?

    A. Isthmus
    B. Corpus
    C. Fundus
    D. Cervix
    E. Body

55. A mature follicle ready for ovulation is referred to as the:

    A. Corpus luteum
    B. Graafian follicle
    C. Corpus albicans
    D. Preantral follicle
    E. Theca lutein

56. Endometrial proliferation is stimulated by:

    A. Human choriogonadotropin
    B. Progesterone
    C. Testosterone
    D. Alpha-fetoprotein
    E. Estrogen

57. Ovarian follicles grow at the daily rate of _____ until ovulation:

    A. 1–2 mm
    B. 2–3 mm
    C. 3–4 mm
    D. 4–5 mm
    E. 5–6 mm

58. FSH is produced by the:

    A. Ovary

B. Corpus luteum

C. Hypothalamus

D. Pituitary

E. Thyroid

59. Which hormone is mostly responsible for premenstrual symptoms and those of early pregnancy?

A. LH

B. FSH

C. Estrogen

D. Progesterone

E. PAPPA

60. Normally, ovulation occurs on which day of the menstrual cycle?

A. 7

B. 14

C. 21

D. 28

E. 30

61. Without fertilization of the ovum, the corpus luteum cyst should regress after:

A. 4 days

B. 8 days

C. 10 days

D. 14 days

62. Precocious puberty in a child could be caused by:

A. Benign cystic teratoma

B. Cystadenoma

C. Arrhenoblastoma

D. Granulose cell tumor

E. Sertoli-Leydig tumor

63. Sonohysterography is a common procedure used to determine some causes of infertility, including:

A. Endometriosis

B. Endometrial polyp

C. Adenomyosis

D. A and B

E. All of the above

64. In vitro fertilization:

A. Permits the physician to retrieve many oocytes

B. Is performed when the tube is not obstructed

C. Allows the physician to retrieve only one oocyte

D. Decreases the number of embryos to be implanted

E. Does not require ultrasound guidance

65. Normally, the endometrium of a postmenopausal patient is usually:

A. Hypoechoic
B. Multi-layered
C. Thick and hyperechoic
D. Thin
E. Cystic

66. Postmenopausal bleeding is most commonly the result of:

A. Benign hyperplasia
B. Endometrial polyps
C. Endometritis
D. Endometrial carcinoma
E. Cervical cancer

67. Extrauterine adnexal masses are most commonly found in the:

A. Ovary
B. Fallopian tubes
C. Cervix
D. Broad ligament
E. Fornix

68. Which of the following characterizes Stein-Leventhal syndrome?

A. Menorrhagia, obesity, and hirsutism
B. Menorrhagia, obesity, and infertility
C. Obesity, hirsutism, and infertility
D. Menorrhagia, hirsutism, and infertility
E. Menorrhagia, obesity, hirsutism, and infertility

69. All of these statements about endometriosis are true EXCEPT:

A. It is a disease of upper middle-class professional women.
B. It is more common among caucasions.
C. There is a hereditary predisposition.
D. Symptoms are cyclic.
E. It is associated with multiparity.

70. Where is a Gartner's duct cyst found?

A. Ovary
B. Uterus
C. Vagina
D. Cervix
E. Broad ligament

71. Noabothian cysts are found in the:

A. Ovary
B. Broad ligament
C. Cervix
D. Vagina
E. Fallopian tube

72. Your patient presents with abdominal swelling, low back pain, and an extremely elevated CA-125. These clinical findings suggest:

A. Pregnancy
B. Infection
C. Hemorrhage
D. Malignancy
E. Findings are nonspecific

73. Perihepatitis can be associated with pelvic inflammatory disease, causing right upper quadrant tenderness and pain. This condition is:

A. PID
B. Fitzhugh-Curtis syndrome
C. Stein-Leventhal syndrome
D. Indistinct uterus
E. Meig's syndrome

74. A patient who has taken oral contraceptives for more than 5 years is at increased risk for developing:

A. Renal cancer
B. Hepatic adenoma
C. Heart disease
D. Lung cancer
E. Ectopic pregnancy

75. Transvaginally, in the sagittal view, the bladder will be seen to fill:

A. In the left lower corner of the image
B. In the right lower corner of the image
C. In the left upper corner of the image
D. In the right upper corner of the image
E. In the middle anterior portion of the image

76. What maneuver would best improve the quality of this longitudinal image through the uterus?

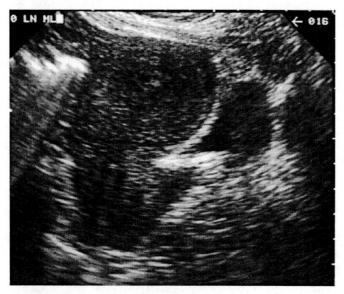

A. Do a transvaginal exam.
B. Adjust TGC.
C. Decrease overall gain.
D. Fill the bladder.
E. Increase overall gain.

77. A disorder that is caused by the presence of only one defective gene is called:

A. Autosomal dominant
B. Autosomal recessive
C. X-linked
D. B and C
E. All of the above

78. Longitudinal and transverse views of the fetal spine are routine on fetal exam. When the normal fetal spine is imaged transversely, the sonogram demonstrates:

A. Two ossification centers positioned an equal distance apart and tapering toward the sacrum
B. Two ossification centers positioned an equal distance apart and splaying outward at the level of the sacrum
C. Three ossification centers, two posterior and one anterior, with the two posterior centers pointing away from each other
D. Three ossification centers, two anterior and one posterior, with the two posterior centers pointing toward each other
E. Three ossification centers, two posterior and one anterior, with the two posterior centers pointing toward each other

79. Perihepatitis can be associated with pelvic inflammatory disease, causing right upper quadrant tenderness and pain. This condition is:

    A. PID

    B. Meigs' syndrome

    C. Fitz-Hugh Curtis syndrome

    D. Stein-Leventhal syndrome

    E. Indistinct uterus

80.   Female pseudohermaphroditism is most often caused by:

    A. Pituitary imbalance

    B. Adrenal hyperplasia

    C. Ovarian masculinization

    D. Testicular feminization

    E. Failure of the mullerian ducts to fuse

81.   Which cardiac abnormality cannot be detected with the four-chamber view?

    A. Complete heart block

    B. Transposition of the great vessels

    C. Cardiomegaly

    D. Hypoplastic left ventricle

    E. Ventricular septal defect

82.   Umbilical cords can vary in length. A cord that appears to be abnormally thickened in an otherwise normal-appearing pregnancy is most likely the result of:

    A. Resistance of blood flow to the fetus

    B. Cord edema

    C. Macrosomia

    D. Vascular duplication of the cord

    E. Excessive Wharton's jelly

83.   To what is the arrow pointing?

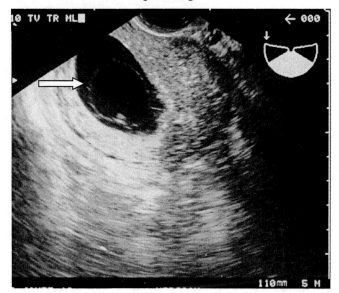

    A. Septum

    B. Chorion

C. Yolk sac

D. Amnion

E. Synechia

84. Of the following choices, the most common cystic mass associated with pregnancy is:

A. Paraovarian

B. Cystadenoma

C. Corpus luteum cyst

D. Follicular cyst

E. Theca lutein cyst

85. Sonographic visualization of a cystic fluid-filled collection adjacent and posterior to the heart most likely represents:

A. Congenital diaphragmatic hernia

B. Pleural effusion

C. Cardiac cyst

D. Aortic aneurysm

E. Cystic adenomatoid malformation

86. Nuchal fold thickness is usually measured at what gestational age?

A. 29–32 weeks

B. 25–28 weeks

C. 22–24 weeks

D. 15–21 weeks

E. 10–14 weeks

87. Lithopedion is:

A. Calcium deficiency

B. Calcified fetus

C. Fetal gallstones

D. Lack of fetal tone

E. Fusion of bone

88. Your patient has a positive pregnancy test and presents with bleeding and cramping. Of the following sonographic findings, which one would make you suspect an inevitable abortion?

A. Dilated cervix

B. Low implantation

C. Irregular sac shape

D. Poor decidual reaction

E. Double yolk sac

89. The purpose of filling the urinary bladder prior to transabdominal ultrasonography includes all of the following EXCEPT:

A. Flattens the uterine angle

B. Provides an acoustic window
C. Provides an internal cystic reference
D. Displaces bowel
E. Magnifies the pelvic organs

90. Large pelvic masses, whether benign or malignant, may cause _____; therefore the _____ should be evaluated also:

    A. Metastatic lesions, liver
    B. Gallstones, gallbladder
    C. Urinary obstruction, kidneys
    D. Biliary obstruction, liver and biliary tree
    E. Portal-splenic hypertension, liver and spleen

91. If a 30-year-old female is on day 8 of her menstrual cycle and she has normal regular periods, her endometrium should measure:

    A. 6 mm
    B. 8 mm
    C. 4 mm
    D. 10 mm
    E. 12 mm

92. For best results, the optimal gestational age for karyotyping by amniocentesis is:

    A. 26–28 weeks
    B. 22–24 weeks
    C. 18–20 weeks
    D. 15–16 weeks
    E. 12–13 weeks

93. A skull that is shaped like a clover leaf is most likely to be associated with:

    A. Thanatophoric dwarfism
    B. Osteogenesis imperfecta
    C. Holoprosencephaly
    D. Spina bifida aperta
    E. Sirenomelia

94. Which of the following lab tests can rule out Down's syndrome in at-risk patients?

    A. Triple screen
    B. Ultrasound
    C. MSAFP
    D. Vesicocentesis
    E. Amniocentesis

95. The terms RVOT (right ventricular outflow tract) and LVOT (left ventricular outflow tract) denote the:

    A. Ascending aorta and inferior vena cava
    B. Descending aorta and pulmonary vein

C. Pulmonary vein and pulmonary artery
D. Pulmonary artery and ascending aorta
E. None of the above

96. A Gartner's duct cyst is found in the:

A. Fallopian tube
B. Cervix
C. Vagina
D. Broad ligament
E. Myometrium

97. The term for absence of menses is:

A. Agenesis
B. Dysmenorrhea
C. Menorrhagia
D. Amenorrhea
E. Metrorrhagia

98. A benign cystic teratoma is commonly found:

A. Posterior and inferior
B. Anterior and superior
C. In the false pelvis
D. In the left adnexa
E. In the right adnexa

99. On physical exam, all of the following would cause a patient to present large for gestational age EXCEPT:

A. Cystadenoma
B. Cystic teratoma
C. Trophoblastic disease
D. Leiomyomas
E. Myometrial contraction

100. Which of the following statements about placental grading is NOT true?

A. A grade III placenta indicates fetal lung maturity.
B. Diabetics often show a grade 0–I at term.
C. Placental grades range from 0–III.
D. Most placentas are grade II at delivery.
E. Placental grading does not reliably predict fetal lung maturation.

101. This image represents which of the following?

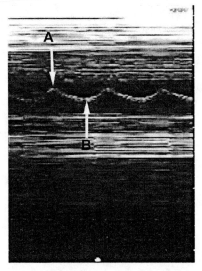

   A. M-mode
   B. D-mode
   C. B-mode
   D. A-mode
   E. PW-mode

102. The lavator ani muscles are seen, transversely, at the same level as the:

   A. Cervix
   B. Uterine corpus
   C. Vagina
   D. Ovaries
   E. Iliac vessels

103. The most common cause of acute postpartum hemorrhage is:

   A. Uterine fibroids
   B. Uterine atony
   C. Endometritis
   D. Succenturiate placenta
   E. Retained products of conception

104. Which of the following statements is NOT true about fetal demise:

   A. Deuel's sign might be present.
   B. Absence of cardiac motion for at least 3 minutes is a sonographic hallmark.
   C. The diagnosis should be confirmed by more than one examiner.
   D. Spalding's sign might be present.
   E. Failure of mother to feel fetal movement is diagnostic

105. Ovulation usually occurs when the dominant follicle reaches the following size:

   A. 1.5 cm
   B. 2.5 cm

C. 3.5 cm

D. 10 mm

E. 15 mm

106. Which of these masses is considered malignant?

A. Endometrioma

B. Dysgerminoma

C. Cystadenoma

D. Dermoid

E. Pyosalpinx

107. The findings in this image of the fetal head strongly suggest:

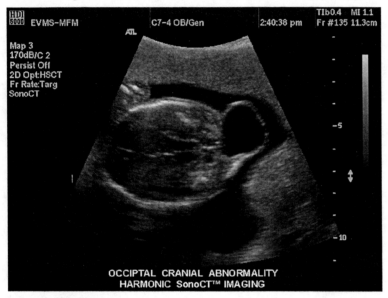

A. Down syndrome

B. Trisomy 13

C. Encephalocele

D. Hydrocephalus

E. Fetal demise

108. Of the following, the most common benign tumor of the uterus is:

A. Leiomyoma

B. Leiomyosarcoma

C. Endometrioma

D. Kruckenburg's

E. Adenomyosa

109. A fetus that weighs 4600 grams at term is said to be:

A. Growth-restricted

B. Post-term

C. Macrosomic

D. Diabetic

E. Small for gestational age (SGA)

110. Corpus luteal cysts accompany early pregnancy and should resolve by:

    A. 8 weeks
    B. 10 weeks
    C. 12 weeks
    D. 14 weeks
    E. 16 weeks

111. Which of the following would not be associated with oligohydramnios?

    A. Intrauterine growth restriction
    B. GI tract obstruction
    C. Intrauterine fetal demise
    D. Premature rupture of membranes
    E. Bilateral renal agenesis

112. A 30-year-old is 1 week postpartum and extremely anemic, exhausted, and just wants to sleep all of the time. You suspect:

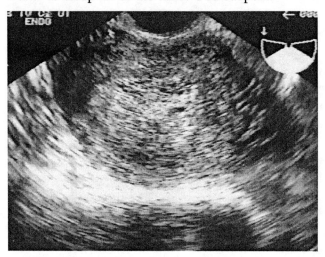

    A. Fibroid uterus
    B. Molar pregnancy
    C. Retained products of conception (RPOC)
    D. Endometrial cancer
    E. Uterine rupture

113. The pelvic mass most commonly seen during a normal first trimester pregnancy is:

    A. Leiomyoma
    B. Theca lutein cysts
    C. Cystic teratoma
    D. Corpus luteal cyst
    E. Cystadenoma

114. When you have demonstrated the fetal stomach transversely at the level of the portal vein, you are at the appropriate level for:

    A. Cord insertion
    B. Fetal kidneys
    C. Three-vessel cord
    D. Thoracic circumference
    E. Abdominal circumference

115. Twin growth is similar to that of singletons up to:

    A. 20 weeks
    B. 30 weeks
    C. 10 weeks
    D. 25 weeks
    E. 15 weeks

116. Which of the following is not associated with holoprosencephaly?

    A. Failure of the cranial vault to form correctly
    B. Failed development of the fetal forebrain
    C. Cyclopia
    D. Proboscis
    E. Fused thalami

117. Choose the statement that most accurately describes the anatomic relationships among the ureter, ovary, and iliac vessels:

    A. The ureter is anterior to the ovary, and the iliac vessels are posterior.
    B. The ureter is posterior to the ovary, and the iliac vessels are anterior.
    C. The ureter and iliac vessels are anterior to the ovary.
    D. The ureter and iliac vessels are posterior to the ovary.
    E. The ureter and iliac vessels are medial to the ovary.

118. Which of the following statements should NOT be written on the technical data sheet?

    A. The uterus is normal in size and shape.
    B. There is fluid noted in the cul-de-sac.
    C. There is an ectopic pregnancy identified in the right adnexa.
    D. The left ovary is enlarged and hypoechoic.
    E. There is no intrauterine pregnancy identified.

119. Which is the best description of micrognathia?

    A. Absence of the nasal septum
    B. Moderate posterior position of the frontal bone
    C. Moderate posterior position of the mandible
    D. Decrease in the normal size of the nasal bone
    E. Decrease in the normal size of the tongue

120. One would not expect to see cul-de-sac fluid with:

    A. Pelvic ascites
    B. Pelvic inflammatory disease
    C. Normal ovulation
    D. Uterine fibroids
    E. Ectopic pregnancy

PART VI

Exam Outline

The American Registry of Diagnostic Medical Sonographers publishes its exam outlines and other important information on its website (www.ARDMS.org). Visit the site for complete information about applying for and taking the registry examinations. The outline for each exam indicates the approximate percentage of the exam that a particular topic represents. This information is important because it indicates the relative importance of each topic and allows you to study more effectively. *Ob/Gyn Sonography Review* covers the material on the revised ARDMS outline.

The complete outline for the Obstetrics and Gynecology specialty examination appears below.

I. Anatomy and Physiology (32%)

    A. Normal Anatomy and Physiology

    B. Perfusion and Function

II. Pathology (32%)

    A. Abnormal Perfusion and Function

    B. Abnormal Physiology

    C. Congenital Anomalies

    D. Pelvic Abnormalities

    E. Placental Abnormalities

III. Integration of Data (7%)

    A. Incorporate outside data

    B. Reporting Results

C. Serial Studies

IV. Protocols (15%)

A. Clinical Standards and Guidelines

B. Measurement Techniques

C. Non-Sonographic Techniques

V. Physics and Instrumentation (9%)

A. Hemodynamics

B. Imaging instruments

VI. Treatment (2%)

A. Sonographer Role in Procedures

PART VII

Bibliography

Obstetrics & Gynecology

//

Benacherraf B: *Ultrasound of Fetal Syndromes*, 2nd edition. New York, Churchill Livingston, 2007.

Berman MC, Cohen HL (eds): *Diagnostic Medical Sonography, A Guide to Clinical Practice—Obstetrics and Gynecology*, 2nd edition. Philadelphia, Lippincott, 1997.

Callen PW (ed): *Ultrasonography in Obstetrics and Gynecology*, 5th edition. Philadelphia, Saunders Elsevier, 2008.*

Curry RA, Tempkin BB (eds): S*onography: Introduction to Normal Structure and Functional,* 3rd edition. St. Louis, Elsevier Saunders, 2011.*

Fleischer AC, Manning FA, Jeanty P, et al (eds): *Sonography in Obstetrics and Gynecology: Principles and Practice*, 7th edition. New York, McGraw-Hill, 2011.

Hagen-Ansert SL (ed): *Textbook of Diagnostic Ultrasonography*, 7th edition. St. Louis, Mosby Elsevier, 2012.*

Henningsen CG: *Clinical Guide to Ultrasonography*, St. Louis, Mosby, 2004.*

Hickey J, Goldberg F: *Ultrasound Review of Obstetrics and Gynecology*. Philadelphia, Lippincott-Raven, 1996.

Reuter K, Babagbemi TK: *Obstetric and Gynecologic Ultrasound: Case Review Series.* St. Louis, Mosby, 2006.

Johnson PT, Kurtz AB: *Case Review: Obstetrical and Gynecologic Ultrasound.* St. Louis, Mosby, 2001.

Rumack CM, Wilson SR, Charboneau JW, et al (eds): *Diagnostic Ultrasound*, 4th edition. St. Louis, Mosby Elsevier, 2010.*

Saunders RC: *Clinical Sonography: A Practical Guide*, 4th edition. Philadelphia, Lippincott, 2006.

Saunders RC: *Clinical Sonography: A Practical Guide*, 3rd edition. Philadelphia, Lippincott, 1998.

Saurbrei EE, Nguyen KT, Nolan RL, et al: *A Practical Guide to Ultrasound in Obstetrics and Gynecology*. Philadelphia, Lippincott-Raven, 1998.

Standring, S: *Gray's Anatomy*, 40th edition. St. Louis, Elsevier/Churchill Livingstone, 2009.*

Ultrasound Physics

Hedrick WR, Hykes DL, Starchman DE: *Ultrasound Physics and Instrumentation*, 4th edition. St.Louis, Elsevier Mosby, 2005.*

Kremkau FW: *Sonography: Principles and Instruments*, 8th edition. Philadelphia, Saunders Elsevier, 2011. *

Kremkau FW: *Diagnostic Ultrasound: Principles and Instruments*, 7th edition. Philadelphia, Saunders Elsevier, 2006.

Owens CA, Zagzebski JA: *Ultrasound Physics Review: SPI Edition*. Pasadena, CA, Davies Publishing, 2009.*

Zagzebski JA: *Essentials of Ultrasound Physics*. St. Louis, Mosby, 1996.*